SUP.ER
eating

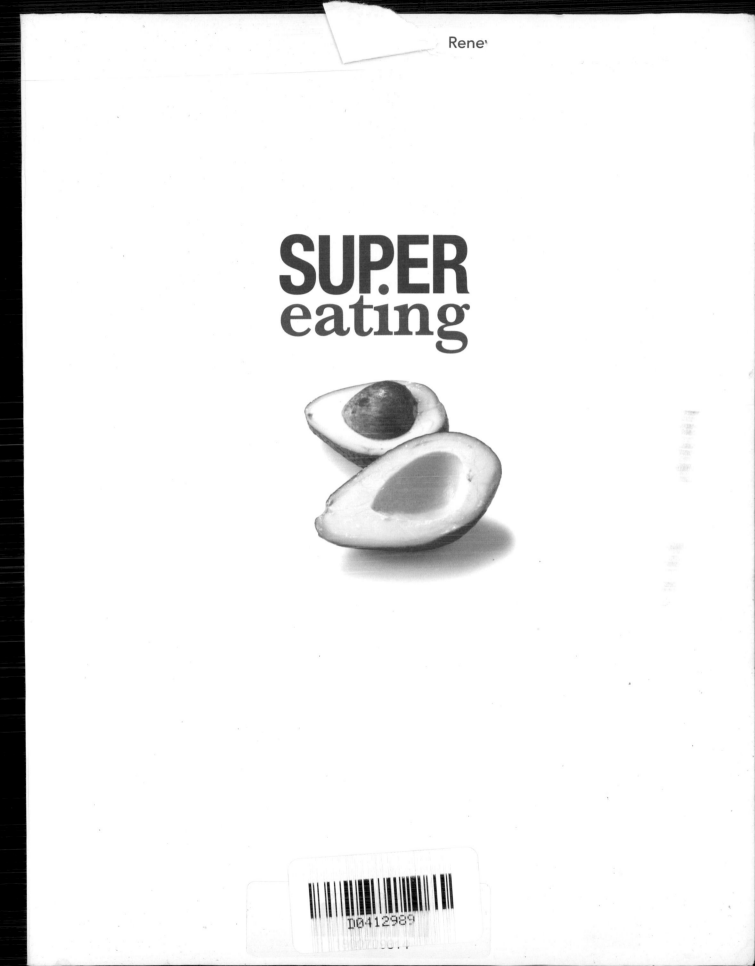

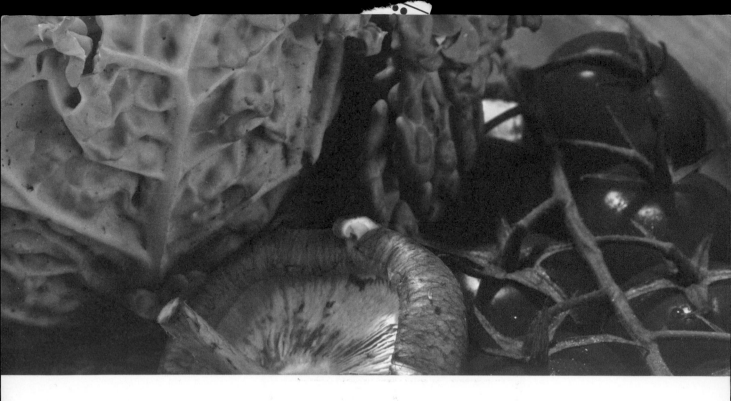

To three great ladies, DSB, SB and JT
with love and appreciation.

IAN MARBER
SUP.ER
eating

a **revolutionary way** to get
more from the **foods you eat**

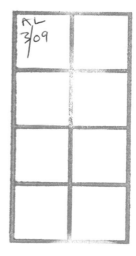

quadrille

Contents

Supereating for Wellbeing 98

How to use the interplay of nutrients to advantage in specific areas of health.

Fighting the ageing process | Boosting the immune system | Dealing with stress
Improving digestive health | Eating for greater energy | Maintaining heart health
Maintaining general skin health | Caring for your joints

Foods for Supereating 146

The nutritional content of a wide range of foods, focusing on the overall effect of the nutrients in each and suggesting which foods can be teamed together to extract maximum goodness from what we eat.

Beans and legumes | Eggs and dairy | Fruit | Fish and seafood | Herbs and spices
Nuts and seeds | Vegetables | Rice and grains | Poultry and lean meats | Others

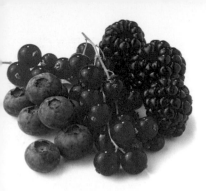

Foreword

Food is one of the few things that bind us together, and the significance of what we eat and how we eat it has come to define nationalities, religions and cultures. Good cooks become celebrated, none more so than the world-famous chefs that dominate in the media, as they show us how it could and should be done. Their creations exude flavour, colour and extravagance, and their recipe books combine foods to enhance the experience of eating.

At the other end of the scale lie the nutrition consultants, dietitians and food gurus who cluck and lecture about what not to eat, with their dire warnings and statistics about painful consequences unless you eat this but don't eat that. The image of the nutritionists is one of science and misery, a far cry from the indulgence and joy that typifies celebrity chefs.

I can see how this has happened, as many nutrition books are filled with advice on how to eat but solely based on looking at food for its constituent parts. The food is deconstructed and reduced to being a collection of nutrients, to help this or do that, with a function and a purpose. Food loses its magic and much of its joyous nature as it is taken apart and left that way.

But this book is about food and still incorporates the joy of eating, together with eating in a way that promotes good health. While it does analyze and deconstruct food, it differs from so many other books of this kind as the food is put back together again. It's about the combination of foods, which ones work together and which ones you should avoid, and is written for those of us who love food but would like it to love us back. The food that we deconstruct ends up intact again as we apply the concept of Supereating to meals and snacks, with no mention of weight, ratio of proteins to carbohydrates or recommended daily allowances of vitamins and minerals.

I love food and I love eating, and I trust that this book reflects that, and not just my interest in nutrition. I also have a passion for cooking but rarely find the time to cook as I might want to, and instead happily cobble together meals. I am aware of what I eat without being overly careful, and, from time to time enjoy the sort of food that my more extreme peers tell me will probably kill me. My favourite meal is probably a fillet steak, plenty of vegetables and some French fries, served with béarnaise sauce and enjoyed with two glasses of a full-bodied Pinot Noir, so I don't fall into the typical eat-well-all-the-time group that perhaps I am expected to.

I am confident that the concept of Supereating has far to go, and that it is a revolutionary way of eating food, not simply ingesting nutrients.

Ian Marber
www.thefooddoctor.com

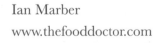

Beyond the
One-step Approach

TO THE UNTRAINED EYE, IT WOULD SEEM THAT NUTRITION HAS COME OF AGE. It has become an accepted part of a healthy lifestyle, and I would argue that it is probably the cornerstone of health. People are aware of what they eat; they talk about it, ask questions of professionals and take advice on ways to tackle common health issues through nutrition. What we feed our children is discussed, argued about and debated by government, in schools, in the home and in the media, and anything short of giving your children organic locally produced food is akin to child-abuse to some. We take supplements, many of them, it seems, in the belief that they can delay the ageing process, prevent disease, allay symptoms and generally make us fitter, slimmer, faster and better.

But, for all this progress, I have often felt that there was something missing, as it all seemed perhaps a little too easy, the information had become almost lightweight. I found that when I was asked for quotes for some magazines and newspapers, the simplest of information had to be made even

"But, for all this progress, I have often felt that there was something missing, as it all seemed perhaps a little too easy, the information had become almost lightweight."

simpler, as if the reader would be confused by anything besides the merest suggestion of changing more than one small thing about their diet. Even the most in-depth and far-reaching of research projects is now reported and communicated to people in simple terms, and so headlines such as 'scientists say that eating X could prevent Y' have become commonplace.

The Next Big Thing

Yet for all this information, there is another level to nutritional advice that has been overlooked, and I feel that until we fully understand this arena, some of the advice we have been given could be limited in its success. In simple terms, the next big thing in nutrition is going to be an increased awareness of the complicated interaction between the nutrients. When we fully understand this relationship – sometimes synergistic as one nutrient will activate or enhance others, sometimes antagonistic as nutrients fight for absorption – then we can truly derive benefit from nutrition.

The Superfoods Shortfall

This idea had been in the background of my mind for some time, unformulated for the most part, but only really surfaced recently when I was writing about the phenomenon of so-called 'superfoods'. For anyone who has managed to avoid the clever marketing of some foods, it seemed to me that, for a while at least, any food that was blessed with a marketing department could happily claim to be a 'superfood'. If a food contained a nutrient that did something, or could prevent, enhance, stop or slow down anything at all, then the food in which this nutrient was found could be categorized as a 'superfood'.

"For anyone who has managed to avoid the clever marketing of some foods, it seemed to me that, for a while at least, any food that was blessed with a marketing department could happily claim to be a 'superfood'."

Seeing as every single nutrient – that is every single vitamin, mineral, essential fatty acid, carotenoid, glucosinolate, organosulphide, phyto-oestrogen or bioflavonoid – does something positive or is involved in some biochemical process that has a positive nature, then surely it could be argued that every food might be a superfood? In practice, however, if the food is a humble vegetable, one without much of a profit margin attached to it, then it is unlikely to have a marketing budget and thus is limited in how its superfood status could be communicated to the public.

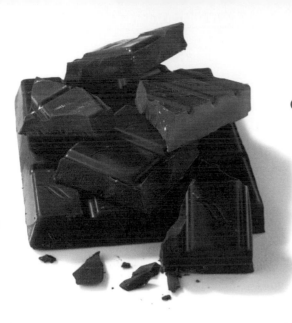

Compare this to dark chocolate, a food that is 'processed' in as much as it is made from other things, not simply grown and sold as is. The manufacturing process allows room for a healthy profit margin, some of which can be spent on marketing. Some bright spark in the press office will realize that the antioxidants found in cocoa beans are just like those in fresh fruits and vegetables and thus the food, in this case chocolate, becomes a 'superfood'. The presence of fat and sugar would be overshadowed by the potential benefits of the antioxidants – in the case of chocolate this would be polyphenols that can protect cells from oxidizing.

In my role as a health journalist, I began to receive dozens of press releases claiming that this food or that food was now a 'superfood' as it could do X or Y. On the face of this, it is not a bad thing to be reminded of the potential that nutrients have, but it was all getting terribly simplistic and my feeling of disquiet increased.

It became most obvious to me when I was asked for a quote for a well-respected glossy magazine. They wanted to know which one food was simply better than the others, which was the 'ultimate superfood'. I couldn't answer, as I understood that no food delivers that – it's the package, the combination, and the reason for this is that the way the nutrients interact is the fine detail that makes the science of nutrition into something powerful, yet until now, it's been 'dumbed down' and overlooked in the interests of making it accessible.

The nutrients we require need to be delivered in a way that encourage as many of them as possible to work together, almost as a team, with a

> **"The nutrients we require need to be delivered in a way that encourage as many of them as possible to work together, almost as a team, with a cohesive strategy rather than allowing any one single nutrient to dominate."**

cohesive strategy rather than allowing any one single nutrient to dominate. In the future, research may show that large amounts of specific nutrients have benefit, indeed they may be vital, but I find it hard to accept that the current thinking of simply shovelling nutrients in via 'superfoods' or supplements with no understanding of how a large amount of one affects the absorption or workings of others is the way we should be thinking about nutrition.

Thus 'Supereating' takes the concept of 'superfoods' further, and, to my mind, to its natural conclusion. Through identifying the relationship between the nutrients, and creating a 'road map' that highlights which ones help each other and which fight or hinder one another, we can create a nutritional protocol that allows us to eat intelligently, not allowing any one nutrient to dominate, but ensuring that the interaction between the entirety of nutrients is enhanced.

Convenience Nutrition

Since I qualified as a nutrition consultant, the cornerstone of my work has been one-to-one consultations. Having begun consulting in 1998, I think I have now completed over 5,000 of these, and I am pleased to report that I learned something each and every time. Whether it has been a better way to communicate a concept, or how to integrate nutrition into a client's life, each consultation has been an experience.

Clients will come to see a nutrition consultant for several reasons, ranging from weight loss to digestion problems, fatigue to hormonal issues, yet one interesting trait that I see again and again is the desire to do the most convenient thing, to find a nutritional solution that involves as little effort as possible, with as little change in beliefs too.

For example, a client with a poor diet may have day-to-day symptoms that they find debilitating, and making dietary changes could bring about a significant improvement in how they feel (after all, that is why they have come to see a nutrition consultant). However, many clients will not make fundamental changes if they are too far removed from what they believe to be true or which involve changing the habits of a lifetime. In other words, they are looking for something that offers rewards with little effort, without being challenged too much (I am not criticizing, merely pointing out an aspect of human behaviour). The matter of convenience is one that is drummed into us time and time again. Everything has to be quick, easy and convenient, which I can understand when it comes to more mundane matters such as supermarket shopping or going to the post office, but I am bemused that we apply the same approach to our health.

> "Everything has to be quick, easy and convenient, which I can understand when it comes to mundane matters such as supermarket shopping or going to the post office, but I am bemused that we apply the same approach to our health."

As we all know, we are now much more aware of our own responsibility in maintaining our own health. The days of being 'under the doctor' are behind us, as we now have access to more of the information about many aspects of health that was hitherto the remit of the family GP. For example, in the past the doctor may have discovered a raised cholesterol level after a routine blood test and recommended that the patient take a statin to address this. Nowadays, we are likely to be aware of a familial trend towards high cholesterol and include some foods in our diet in an effort to avoid taking medication. However, much of the advice we get on how to improve our diet these days comes from the people that sell us the food, and it could well be argued that they have a vested interest in manipulating information so that their products provide the answer.

> "However, much of the advice we get on how to improve our diet these days comes from the people that sell us the food, and it could well be argued that they have a vested interest in manipulating information so that their products provide the answer."

For example, rather than take a statin, many people choose to use a growing range of functional foods, in this case spreads and yoghurts made with plant sterols that lower cholesterol. There are other measures that could be adopted, such as reducing the intake of saturated fats, increasing fibre in the diet by including foods that contain beta-glucans, specifically oats, and exercising on a regular basis. But these would need to be consistently included, and require some effort, certainly more than just adding in one serving of a functional yoghurt every day.

The One-step Approach

This approach, the simple, easy one is something I call the 'One-step Approach'. It's one step away from the problem, requires little effort and delivers some (often limited) results, and it doesn't require any major change in thinking, so isn't too challenging. The results could well be a lot better if we put more into it, but the investment seems worthy of the reward, and all too often we are complacent, so we stick to the easy route.

I feel we use the same One-step Approach when it comes to a variety of health issues:

Got a headache? Take aspirin.

Joint pain? An anti-inflammatory should do the trick.

Now, when we apply the same theory to nutrition we can take the same simplistic approach. We tend to think of nutrients in a linear way, in other words vitamin X does Y and is found in Z. Therefore, if we work out that we need more X we should eat more Z. Simple. But is it too simple? What have we lost along the way by simplifying the information? Is the result therefore compromised?

Most of us are familiar with vitamin C, and we know a few things about what it does. Generally, most people seem to think, rightly or wrongly, that vitamin C helps cure or speed up recovery from the common cold, and is found in citrus fruits. So if you have a cold, drink orange juice. It's familiar, simple and a classic example of a One-step Approach. It's not wrong, but there is more to the story.

So, got a cold? Take vitamin C.

Constipated? Take magnesium.

Need more calcium... ? Eat more…

Now, I am prepared to make a bet here. Did you think 'dairy products' then? Or just milk? Of course you did, because we have been told time and time again that dairy products contain calcium (indeed they do) and that calcium is required for bone density (and it is). So what's wrong with this? In essence, it's correct, but if you are someone who has been told that osteoporosis is a risk, is eating more dairy products the answer or is it a One-step Approach that over-simplifies the situation to make things easy?

> "If you are someone who has been told that osteoporosis is a risk, is eating more dairy the answer or is it a One-step Approach that over-simplifies the situation to make things easy?"

I maintain that we can make a significant improvement in our overall nutrition only by taking the more complex, yet ultimately more beneficial approach that is Supereating.

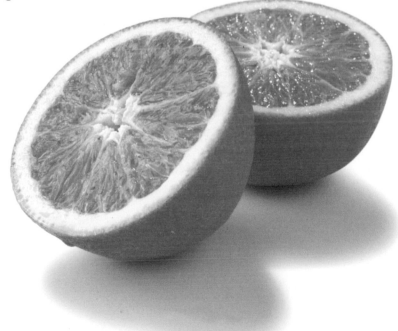

TOWARDS THE SUPEREATING APPROACH

Using the bone density example, let me explain the principles of Supereating as simply as possible. If you eat more dairy produce to get the calcium, as we have all been encouraged to do, what else might happen as a result of this increased consumption? Will your intake of saturated fats increase accordingly and thus potentially contribute to cholesterol issues? Is the calcium in dairy produce right for you, and if it is could it be better absorbed by combining the chosen source of calcium with another food? Is there a source of calcium that delivers other benefits too, such as dark green leafy vegetables that contain fibre? Also, for the calcium to be absorbed into the bone efficiently we need magnesium, so what is the correct ratio of magnesium to calcium, and having established that, what foods deliver that ratio?

It's a challenging and exciting area of nutrition that has hitherto been largely ignored, but the relationship between nutrients is an important aspect of good nutrition, and I will show you how combining specific foods can help you get the very best from your food to deliver a level of nutritional health that surpasses what we have previously understood. We will look at the relationship between the nutrients, which ones help and which hinder absorption, together with the role that probiotics play in the synthesis of some nutrients. I will show you how to put together an eating plan for specific conditions that offers the ultimate delivery of nutrients, so that old-fashioned eating becomes Supereating, thus changing the way you eat for good.

> "I will show you how combining specific foods can help you get the very best from your food to deliver a level of nutritional health that surpasses what we have previously understood. "

There are many relationships between nutrients but not all of them are relevant to human nutrition. Of those that are, the interactions that take place between them tend to occur in the large intestine. The studies that have been carried out on these interactions usually focus on two or three nutrients, but in reality, every time we eat we ingest food that contains a very wide range of nutrients, and so it is the relationship between all the nutrients that is actually of more interest.

However, research into this is limited as it would be almost impossible to assess fully how all the nutrients interact in the human body. Interestingly, some of the interactions are mutual, while others are one-directional. The ones that have a mutual relationship are those that have similar chemical structures and absorption routes. Therefore minerals will tend to have mutual relationships with other minerals and vitamins with other vitamins.

There are three types of relationships between the nutrients:

✔ The nutrients have a mutual effect on one another, i.e. each influences the action or absorption of the other.

● One nutrient remains passive as the other affects its action.

✗ A third party substance influences the activity or absorption of the nutrients.

Supereating examines these three types of nutritional relationships and offers a solution to get the best from food by combining it in a way that encourages synergy and harmony between the nutrients.

The Limitations of Supplementation

I am often baffled by the level of supplementation that some people favour. In many ways, taking vitamin and mineral supplements is the ultimate in the One-step Approach as the most simplistic of theories is applied. I am totally in favour of supplementation where it is appropriate, but I do feel that many health professionals who use supplements to effect a change do not consider the wider implications of their actions on the other nutrients.

Furthermore, when taking a supplement to bring about a change, we have to ask how long we take it for and whether such long-term use could have any side effects. For example, a woman of 25 experiencing menstrual cramping may be recommended to take a supplement of magnesium shortly before her period. This should alleviate the discomfort. Assuming, however, that she menstruates for another 25 years, is she to take the supplement every month, or 300 times? Will her zinc levels be affected? Are her calcium levels a consideration? If so, is it still worth taking the magnesium supplement, or is there another way of encouraging higher magnesium intake and absorption without the potential side effect?

It must be said that the simplistic One-step Approach to supplementation is a factor that we need to be aware of. There are many health issues that can be addressed by taking supplements of a single nutrient. For example, zinc has many roles, and is often recommended by nutrition professionals as a measure to enhance fertility in both sexes. However, increased protein in the diet can enhance zinc absorption, and unless the food you are eating contains no zinc, which is almost impossible, then changing the ratio of protein to carbohydrates in the diet could be a more favourable answer. If zinc is taken in isolation, then this could affect iron uptake. Added to which calcium absorption could be adversely affected. So, potentially solving one problem creates others in its wake.

"The trick is to enhance absorption at all times, ensuring the various elements of each meal and snack are taken into account. This could be as simple as adding lemon juice (for its citric acid) to vegetables to increase iron absorption."

The trick is to enhance absorption at all times, ensuring the various elements of each meal and snack are taken into account. This could be as simple as adding lemon juice (for its citric acid) to vegetables to increase iron absorption. It is interesting to note that some elements can inhibit the absorption of nutrients even though they are required by the body and increased intake of them has many benefits. For example, polyphenols found in a wide variety of fresh produce are a type of antioxidant that can potentially slow the ageing process have a role to play in preventing the formation of cancerous cells and protect against cardiovascular disease. Polyphenols are found in red wine and olive oil, and it is these that give these foods their healthy reputation. However, polyphenols can inhibit the absorption of iron, and so we have to weigh up which is of more importance, or, better still, offset the inhibition by including an element to enhance absorption. I am not suggesting that you add lemon juice to red wine, but you could ensure that the meal the wine accompanies contains lemon juice or plain yoghurt as the latter contains lactic acid that has the same effect as citric acid. By the way, red wine can also enhance zinc absorption, so that's another factor we need to be aware of.

The Balanced View

It's obviously a complicated area, and the overall benefits of increased absorption have to be considered in relation to the potential downside. I will take all this into account when recommending the combinations of food throughout the book, but there is no doubt that some of the most subtle changes can bring about improvements to most diets.

The research that supports the Supereating approach is available at www.thefooddoctor.com

Supereating
Guide to Nutrients

A NUTRIENT IS ANYTHING THAT WE DERIVE FROM THE ENVIRONMENT that is necessary for us to live and grow, mostly food and water. The nutrients we are most familiar with are vitamins and minerals. There are, however, several other substances found in food that are considered nutrients, including probiotics, essential fatty acids (EFAs) and phytochemicals, or plant chemicals, which are not vital but have powers to promote good health.

The accepted view of nutrients is that they are a 'good thing' and the more the better, as increased nutrient intake means better nutrition, which equals better health. As you will have seen in Chapter 1, the aim of Supereating is to promote the best nutrition possible through a combination of nutrients that complement one another rather than focussing on the few, as by eating foods that deliver nutrients in a positive ratio we can achieve a far better level of nutrition. After all, that's how we eat, with a combination of foods delivering different nutritional elements as a package, not just in one food but in snacks and meals.

In this chapter, all the nutrients are explained in detail, including what they are, a little bit of their history and how they are used by the body. Then we go into more depth exploring the Supereating element, which identifies the nutrient's 'friends' and 'foes'. For example, staying with perhaps the best-known nutrient, calcium, like all nutrients it has friends that promote its absorption and utilization, and foes that block its absorption or increase the demand for this specific nutrient. On pages 50–51 you will see that calcium's absorption is affected by three key factors. One is low levels of hydrochloric acid in the stomach, but the other two relate directly to foods; both phytates and oxalates can hinder the absorption of calcium from food. Phytates are found in grains, beans, legumes, nuts and seeds, many of which contain calcium anyway, but the phytate content reduces its availability. Oxalates are found in some soft fruits, the grain quinoa, almonds and peanuts, amongst other foods. Given our basic knowledge of calcium, i.e. that dairy products are their best sources, what happens when we eat a calcium-rich food with a food rich in phytates? Absorption is reduced, so we counteract this with the friends. Supereating would give maximum uptake and utilization of the mineral by ensuring the presence of vitamin D, magnesium, inulin, potassium and probiotics.

Vitamin A is actually a

generic term covering several different but related compounds. These fat-soluble vitamins are also known collectively as retinoids. We can also make our own vitamin A from a group of nutrients called carotenoids, which are found mainly in red-, orange- and yellow-coloured fruits and vegetables. Beta-carotene, the orange pigment in carrots, is probably the best known of these.

What are the best food sources?

The most concentrated source of vitamin A is in liver (from meat, poultry and fish), but eggs, cheese and yoghurt are also good. Carrots, sweet potato, squash, broccoli, peppers, avocado, peaches, apricots, melon, mangoes and papayas are good vegetarian sources.

✔ Friends

• **Dietary fat and animal protein** can improve vitamin A absorption and utilization.
• **Zinc:** low levels of this mineral appear to depress vitamin A levels.
• **Iron:** low levels of iron also depress vitamin A levels.

✘ Foes

Conditions that compromise the absorption of fat and can lead to vitamin A deficiency:

• **Crohn's and coeliac disease** both compromise fat absorption.
• **Compromised liver and gall bladder function** can result in depressed levels of vitamin A.
• **Very-low-fat diets.**
• **Very-low-protein diets** will disrupt vitamin transport and utilization because these pathways are protein-dependent.
• **Cholesterol-lowering 'functional foods'.**

SEE ALSO
_____

Iron *p58*   Zinc *p74*   **Boosting the Immune System** *p106*   **Maintaining General Skin Health** *p136*

How does the body use it?

Vitamin A has a huge variety of functions in the body, from eye health to the reproductive system. We know the old wives' tale about carrots and seeing in the dark, but like most tales it does carry some scientific weight as vitamin A is active in the synthesis of the rod cells that adapt the eyes to function in low-light conditions (indeed the term retinoid comes from retina).

This vitamin is also extremely important for the immune system: it supports the thymus in the production of white blood cells as well as regulating the activation of specific immune cells; it is an active antioxidant and it plays a role in the formation of all our mucous membranes, which are the first line of defence for our entire body from the gastrointestinal tract to the eyes, ears and lungs. Vitamin A also has mild anti-viral properties.

Vitamin A is essential for a healthy reproductive system in both men and women, playing a role in genetic regulation and promoting normal bone metabolism, as well as cell growth and development. It also works with iron in the formation of red blood cells.

Vitamin A also plays a role in sebum production and is a potent antioxidant, so is therefore important for healthy-looking skin.

WHAT ARE THE SIGNS OF GETTING TOO LITTLE?
Not surprisingly, poor immune function, viral infections and respiratory problems can all be signs of vitamin A deficiency. Acne and other skin conditions, such as goose-bump-like symptoms on the arms and thighs, can be related to deficiency.

Eye conditions, particularly dry eyes, can be signs of vitamin A deficiency. Poor hair and weak nails are other possible signs.

IS IT POSSIBLE TO GET TOO MUCH?
Care needs to be taken during pregnancy not to ingest excess vitamin A as this can be toxic to the foetus. Vitamin A over-stimulates cell proliferation, which can cause birth defects.

Excess vitamin A can also cause liver damage as well as bone pain, but these are usually associated with very large doses taken as supplements.

A day's Supereating

BREAKFAST
live full-fat yoghurt, fresh apricots (or dried apricots that have been soaked overnight), papayas and ground pecan nuts

LUNCH
salad of grated raw carrot and sweet potato with feta cheese, scattered with soya nuts

DINNER
mackerel with a squash risotto and broccoli

Vitamin C,

with the possible exception of calcium, must be the best-known and certainly the most widely supplemented nutrient. Also known as ascorbic acid, vitamin C is a water-soluble vitamin and one that human beings – unlike most other mammals – cannot make for themselves. As hunter-gatherers, our diets would have been quite high in vitamin C, but the modern Western diet is probably not providing the same levels, although there is some disagreement as to whether we actually need quite so much.

We need a vitamin C intake from our food or other sources of at least 300mg daily, which is the equivalent of perhaps 6 average-sized oranges. As it's also found in many other foods, a serious deficiency of vitamin C is rare these days.

Worldwide seagoing exploration historically owes as much to this vitamin as it does to the invention of accurate instruments. Until the link between scurvy and vitamin C deficiency was discovered in 1747, a sailor was about 200 times more likely to die of this disease than enemy action; sadly it took another half century for the naval and medical establishments to recognize the importance of fruit for the sailors' diet.

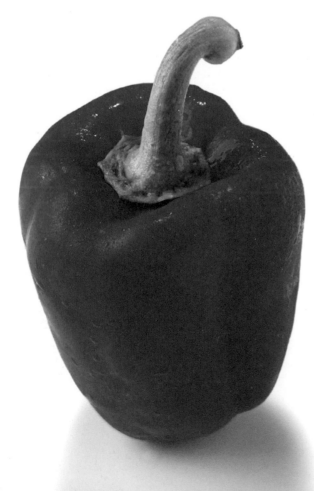

✔ Friends

• Surprisingly, it doesn't seem to have any, although current research seems to indicate that **bioflavonoids** might help absorption.

✗ Foes

• Because vitamin C is so easily excreted, less than ideal levels may be common, particularly for those who drink a great deal of water.
• **Infections** use up higher than normal quantities, as does **smoking**.
• **Cooking** destroys vitamin C, so a proportion of raw fruit and vegetables should be eaten daily.

SEE ALSO
Vitamin E *p28*   Iron *p58*   Bioflavonoids *p76*   Boosting the Immune System *p106*   Dealing with Stress *p112*
Maintaining Heart Health *p128*   Maintaining General Skin Health *p136*

How does the body use it?

Vitamin C is used in incredibly diverse ways, but is probably most commonly recognized for its role in our immune system, where it promotes resistance to infection, whether bacterial or viral. It is also an important free-radical-scavenging antioxidant and it works closely with vitamin E, another important antioxidant vitamin.

Vitamin C is vital for healthy connective tissue because it is used in the formation of collagen, hence its role in preventing scurvy and ensuring healthy skin. Healthy tendons, ligaments and bone structure are all dependent on vitamin C, as is effective wound healing.

Cardiovascular health relies on vitamin C not only for healthy blood vessel walls, but also for preventing oxidative damage to blood fats.

Vitamin C helps to combat stress because it is used in the formation of adrenal hormones.

High vitamin C levels in a meal can help promote the absorption of iron.

WHAT ARE THE SIGNS OF GETTING TOO LITTLE?

Poor immunity, particularly a susceptibility to colds, is an early sign of vitamin C deficiency.

The breakdown of collagen is another sign, so bleeding gums, easy bruising and poor wound healing can indicate low levels.

IS IT POSSIBLE TO GET TOO MUCH?

Very high levels of supplementation can lead to temporary gastrointestinal disturbances.

What are the best food sources?

Vitamin C is found in all fresh fruit and vegetables, but particularly good sources include acerola cherries, all citrus fruits, cantaloupe melons, pineapples, blackcurrants, strawberries, kiwi fruit, peppers, potatoes, sweet potatoes, cauliflower and dark green leafy vegetables such as kale.

A day's Supereating

BREAKFAST
smoothie of cantaloupe melon and mixed berries, with yoghurt and crushed seeds

LUNCH
small baked jacket potato with a salad of broccoli florets and red peppers

DINNER
duck breast with cherries and shredded kale lightly wilted with garlic and onion, and orange wedges

Vitamin D

Vitamin D is a fat-soluble vitamin that is available to us in two ways: we can form our own vitamin D and we can obtain it from food. The way we make our own vitamin D is interesting, because it is not at all straightforward. Cholesterol in our skin reacts with ultraviolet light to make an inactive form of vitamin D, which is then carried to the liver to be activated. This is the most prevalent form of the vitamin, found circulating in our blood. But that's not the end of the story, as vitamin D is further transformed to its most potent form in the kidney. This same pathway is also needed to convert ingested vitamin D. Calcitriol is the name given to activated vitamin D. Plants make vitamin D in much the same way, using their own form of steroid called egosterol.

What are the best food sources?

Vitamin D is found naturally in very few foods, but oily fish provide significant levels. Soya products can provide vitamin D and shiitake mushrooms are also a very good source. Egg yolks provide low levels. Vitamin D is also found in fortified foods, such as breakfast cereals, but these tend to be highly processed and contain too much salt and sugar to be healthy. It is also found in margarines, although these are also perhaps not the best choice.

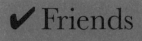
✔ Friends

- **Sunshine** is vital for vitamin D synthesis in the skin.

✗ Foes

The major cause of vitamin D deficiency is low exposure to sunlight. This can be a major factor for several groups:

- **Women whose ethnic culture requires forms of dress that cover their skin at all times**.
- Those living in **low sunlight areas**, particularly in northern latitudes: for example bone mineralization decreases during the winter in Finland.
- **People with dark skins living away from tropical regions**, as they may not get sufficiently strong sunlight to form vitamin D.
- **The use of sunscreen, even at levels as low as factor 15,** can suppress vitamin D formation in the skin.

- The ability to make vitamin D in the skin declines with **age** and this may be combined with reduced exposure to sunlight.
- **Obesity** can disrupt vitamin D levels, firstly because fat cells store vitamin D effectively locking it away and, secondly, because fat cells may compromise the formation of vitamin D in the skin.
- **An imbalance in dietary fat**, such as that due to very-low-fat diets, can disrupt the absorption of dietary vitamin D.
- **Fat malabsorption** due to various factors: liver or gall bladder problems, functional foods that reduce fat absorption.

How does the body use it?

Vitamin D was only discovered in 1920, when its importance for bone structure was first recognized, but ongoing research is fast uncovering a much broader range of influence.

It is important for the health of bones and teeth for several reasons, it is vital for calcium absorption in the gut and can prevent the loss of calcium in urine. The vitamin also acts in a similar way to maintain levels of phosphorus, another important bone mineral.

Vitamin D has now been shown to be very important for maintaining our immune defences, stimulating our basic immune responses while preventing inappropriate immune reactions such as rhinitis and eczema. It may also be protective from some forms of cancer, particularly breast cancer.

Vitamin D plays a role in maintaining blood sugar balance and is also connected to the mechanisms that regulate blood pressure.

WHAT ARE THE SIGNS OF GETTING TOO LITTLE?

Sadly, studies show that vitamin D deficiency is increasingly common, being prevalent across all age groups, ethnic groups and seasons.

The most familiar signs of vitamin D deficiency are linked to bone health, conditions such as rickets in children and osteomalacia (or bone softening) in adults. Osteoporosis can also be caused by low levels of the vitamin, while muscle weakness is another linked symptom.

Inappropriate immune responses such as eczema, allergic rhinitis and even lupus may be linked to low vitamin D.

IS IT POSSIBLE TO GET TOO MUCH?

Excess vitamin D supplementation over many months may cause problems such as diarrhoea or constipation, headache, loss of appetite, nausea and excess circulating levels of calcium. Kidney stones can also form as calcium is deposited in the kidneys, and no more than 1,000iu daily from all sources is recommended. However, studies are suggesting that the current recommended daily intakes of 200–600iu for adults are low and amounts in excess of 700iu are necessary for prevention of fracture in post-menopausal women.

A day's Supereating

BREAKFAST
smoked salmon with scrambled egg

LUNCH
seafood salad in a good olive oil dressing

DINNER
grilled sardines with mixed roast vegetables drizzled in olive oil

Note: the oily dressings will help with the absorption of the vitamin D and if you eat these meals outside in the sun, you will be obtaining even more of this important nutrient

Vitamin E is a generic term for a group of fat-soluble vitamins. These are divided into two related families, tocopherol and tocotrienol, that each have four different forms, alpha, beta, gamma and delta. Vitamin E is found mainly in its alpha-tocopherol form. Because vitamin E is fat-soluble, it can be stored in the body, where it is found in the blood, brain, sex organs (male and female), liver and skin.

Historically, research into vitamin E has focussed on alpha and gamma tocopherol, consequently the tocotrienols have largely been overlooked. Very recent research, however, suggests that all forms of vitamin E are significantly active, each with their own defined roles.

What are the best food sources?

Wheat germ provides excellent levels of vitamin E. Vegetable and olive oils are also good sources, with wheat germ, sunflower, borage seed and almond oils coming out best. Sunflower seeds provide excellent levels of vitamin E; almonds, hazelnuts and peanuts provide reasonable levels, as do avocados and sun-dried tomatoes. With the exception of spinach and Swiss chard, green vegetables do not provide significant amounts of vitamin E. Similarly, fruit is not high in vitamin E, although dried apricots provide low levels. Oily fish, notably tuna, can provide some vitamin E.

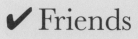

✔ Friends

- **Vitamin C** works very closely with vitamin E by helping to recycle it, making it more effective.
- **Selenium** enhances the uptake of vitamin E.
- Studies suggest that the vitamin E family works synergistically, so all forms should be taken as a whole. Food sources will provide this important mix.

✗ Foes

Conditions that compromise the absorption of fat can lead to vitamin E deficiency:

- **Crohn's and coeliac disease** both compromise fat absorption.
- **Very-low-fat diets.**
- **Cholesterol-lowering 'functional foods'.**
- Other factors include **the processing of vegetable oils to give them shelf life**, which not only compromises vitamin content of the food but also increases demand for vitamin E as an antioxidant.
- **Smoking** increases the body's demand for vitamin E.
- Vitamin E can only be carried around the body once it has been 'activated' by the liver, so **poor liver function** will compromise availability.

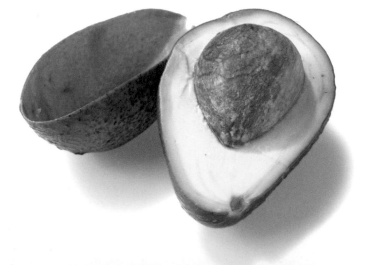

SEE ALSO

Vitamin A *p22*   Vitamin C *p24*   Vitamin B12 *p46*   Selenium *p68*   Boosting the Immune System *p106*
Maintaining Heart Health *p128*   Maintaining General Skin Health *p136*

How does the body use it?

Vitamin E is most widely recognized for its antioxidant activity, where it acts to protect fats from free radical damage. This has wide-ranging implications for health, putting vitamin E in the first line of defence against a long list of conditions: it reduces the damage from high cholesterol by preventing the build-up of plaque on the arterial walls and by thinning the blood, thereby protecting against heart disease and stroke; it reduces the risk of cataract formation in the eye; it works in the skin to protect it from damage due to exposure to ultraviolet light; it appears to be protective against various cancers, including that of the lung, breast and prostate. Because vitamin E is protective against damage to fats there is also evidence that it can slow the progression of Alzheimer's disease.

Vitamin E is extremely important during the early stages of life, from the time of conception to the postnatal development of the infant. Significant levels cross the placenta to the foetus and very high levels in colostrums (beestings, 'first milk' or 'immune milk') provide the infant with antioxidant protection.

Other research suggests that vitamin E can increase immunity, particularly in the elderly, and it has been used to alleviate premenstrual breast pain and tenderness.

Vitamin E appears to have a beneficial effect on selenium levels, is needed for the utilization of vitamin B12 and is involved in the transfer of chemical information from cell to cell.

Vitamin E can also be used topically to soothe skin conditions such as sunburn and to promote healing and reduce scarring.

WHAT ARE THE SIGNS OF GETTING TOO LITTLE?
Not surprisingly, signs of deficiency of vitamin E are linked to increased free radical damage, such as cataracts, angina and other cardiovascular symptoms, as well as damage to peripheral nerves. Dry skin could also denote low levels of vitamin E.

IS IT POSSIBLE TO GET TOO MUCH?
Excessive vitamin E supplementation can lead to easy bruising and bleeding as well as affect blood clotting. Vitamin E can also deplete vitamin A if ingested in excessive amounts.

A day's Supereating

BREAKFAST
porridge (for its selenium) sprinkled with wheat germ, almonds and sunflower seeds and soaked apricots; glass of freshly squeezed orange juice (to provide vitamin C)

LUNCH
shredded spinach salad with avocados and a dressing made from cold-pressed sunflower oil

DINNER
grilled sardines with rice (more selenium) and a green salad tossed in a cold-pressed sunflower oil dressing and scattered with toasted sunflower seeds; follow with a small fruit salad (for more vitamin C)

Vitamin K is a fat-soluble

vitamin found in two different forms: those that are obtained directly from food sources and those manufactured by gut bacteria. It is rather like vitamin D in as much as we have the ability to produce more of our own vitamin K than we obtain from our diets, although not enough for optimal function, so some vitamin K from the diet is considered essential.

Vitamin K was first identified in Denmark in the 1930s, when bleeding was discovered in chicks fed on a fat-free diet. This link with blood clotting gave vitamin K its name (from *koagulation*).

The dietary form of vitamin K is called phylloquinone, while the vitamin K compounds manufactured by our own gut bacteria are called menaquinones.

We store very little vitamin K, but the body compensates for this by recycling what we do have, making the process quite efficient.

✔ Friends

• **Healthy gut bacteria**.
• Foods that contain **good levels of probiotics** (100 million per gram is ideal but over 10 million is good).
• **Prebiotics**, or foods that contain **insoluble fibre** to nourish gut bacteria (found in pulses, grains and vegetables).

✗ Foes

• The major cause of low vitamin K levels is **poor gut bacteria levels**, which could be due to long term use of antibiotics or a high-sugar diet.
• Because of its method of activation, **liver disease** could result in low vitamin K function.
• **Salicylates**, mainly found in aspirin, may inhibit vitamin K recycling.
• As with all fat-soluble vitamins, a **low-fat diet** and **functional foods that inhibit fat absorption** may suppress vitamin K levels.

What are the best food sources?

The best food source of vitamin K is green leafy vegetables, particularly broccoli, kale and Swiss chard, peppers, squash and tomatoes. Parsley is very high in vitamin K, but you would need to eat several spoonfuls. Vitamin K is also present in olive oil, rapeseed oil and soybean oil.

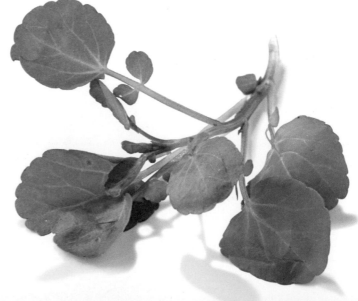

Probiotics *p86*   **Dealing with Stress** *p112*   **Maintaining Heart Health** *p128*

How does the body use it?

Having been identified for its role in clotting, vitamin K perhaps remains best-known for that function. This nutrient single-handedly sets in motion a series of events called 'the coagulation cascade', which refers to the activation by the liver of seven clotting factors each of which is needed to stop bleeding when we are wounded.

Research into vitamin K is ongoing, but there is evidence that it is activated in every cell of the body and plays a role in the development and ageing of the nervous system, particularly the brain. Vitamin K has been found in bone-forming cells, so plays a role in maintaining healthy bones. It is also present in blood vessels, where it may prevent the build up of plaque on the arterial walls. It may also play a role in cancer prevention, due to its cell-signalling abilities. Research into all these aspects of vitamin K is ongoing and there is still much to discover about this important vitamin.

WHAT ARE THE SIGNS OF GETTING TOO LITTLE?

Deficiency is rare, due to our ability to make vitamin K in the gut. If levels do fall, the first signs are linked to its clotting ability, so easy bruising and problems with bleedings such as nose bleeds, heavy menstrual bleeding and blood in the stool may denote vitamin K deficiency. Laboratory tests that measure clotting can be used to assess deficiency.

Problems with bone density could be related to low levels of vitamin K.

Infants may be in danger of low vitamin K levels, particularly premature babies, because their gut is sterile and therefore not producing any vitamin K. This is perfectly natural, but could become a problem if there are any difficulties at birth or if there is the need for surgery.

IS IT POSSIBLE TO GET TOO MUCH?

It is difficult to get too much vitamin K from food and our internal production is regulated by requirement. High doses are not toxic but could cause problems when combined with an anti-coagulant medication such as Warfarin.

There has been speculation that green tea may raise levels of vitamin K, but the amount of tea that would need to be drunk for any measurable result is so high (over 200 cups) that this is not conceivably a problem.

A day's Supereating

REAKFAST
live yoghurt (to promote good gut bacteria), with mixed flake cereal (to provide plenty of prebiotics) and fresh fruit

LUNCH
watercress, spinach and parsley soup with wholemeal bread (to provide prebiotics)

DINNER
stir-fried chicken with red peppers, broccoli and artichoke hearts, drizzled with olive oil (artichoke hearts are high in inulin, a very good prebiotic)

Vitamin B1, also known

as thiamine, is so-called because it was the first B vitamin to be discovered, back in the 1930s. Water-soluble, like all the other members of the B family, it is found in high concentrations in skeletal muscle, the heart, liver, kidneys and brain.

What are the best food sources?

Whole grains and wholewheat pasta, lentils and beans provide reasonable levels of thiamine, but the highest levels can be found in wheat germ, sunflower seeds and lean pork.

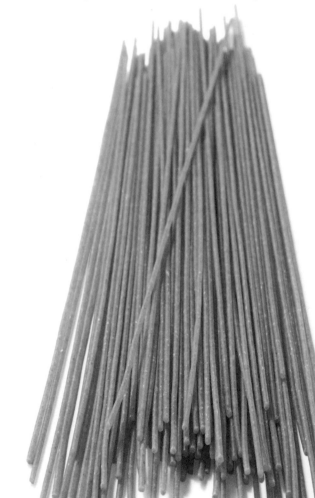

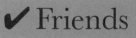
✔ Friends

• Other **B vitamins** are important because they work in synergy.
• Daily consumption of **live yoghurt** can increase levels of thiamine.
• **Magnesium** is important, allowing thiamine to be used in several of its enzymatic actions.

✘ Foes

• The major cause of low thiamine in the West is **high alcohol intake**.
• Long-term use of **water-retention medication** can deplete thiamine levels.
• **Food processing**, such as the polishing of rice, can remove all thiamine.
• Some foods can inactivate thiamine, such as **tea and coffee when drunk in large amounts**.
• Some foods break down thiamine too quickly, particularly **raw fish**. This would mean that someone relying on sushi as a staple of their diet could risk low thiamine levels.
• **Cooking at high temperatures** can inactivate thiamine and it will be lost into the cooking liquid.

SEE ALSO

Other B vitamins *pp34–47*   **Magnesium** *p60*   **Probiotics** *p86*   **Improving Digestive Health** *p118*
Eating for Greater Energy *p124*   **Maintaining Heart Health** *p128*

How does the body use it?

In common with all the B family of vitamins, thiamine works closely with other family members. It is primarily required in the cycle of reactions needed to make energy. Thiamine is used as an enzyme in reactions to turn both glucose and fats into energy and for the storage of fats.

Thiamine is important for maintaining a healthy cardiovascular system and may slow the progression of heart disease. It is also vital for a healthy nervous system and nerve communication, so may have a role to play in boosting memory. It is particularly important during pregnancy and soon after birth. As alcohol depletes thiamine levels, drinking alcohol during pregnancy can have a serious effect on foetal brain development.

Thiamine is also important for digestion, partly because it is needed for making the energy required to digest foods and partly because it is needed to produce digestive hydrochloric acid in the stomach.

Thiamine is often recommended as an insect repellent, for both topical and internal use. More research is needed to assess its efficacy in this respect, although many people do report that taking a B complex supplement before travelling to hot climates does reduce the incidence of mosquito bites.

WHAT ARE THE SIGNS OF GETTING TOO LITTLE?
The most widely recognized sign of severe thiamine deficiency is a disease called beriberi. This disease is not usually apparent in the West as it is linked to diets based on polished rice, the processing of which removes many vital nutrients, including thiamine.

Sadly, alcohol-related thiamine deficiency can affect anyone.

The symptoms of vitamin B1 deficiency mirror those systems that are dependent on adequate levels. Fatigue and muscle weakness reflect low energy production; irritability, confusion, depression and tingling nerves result from low thiamine function in the nervous system; rapid heartbeat and sweating could be cardiovascular signs of low thiamine; indigestion, poor nutrient absorption and weight loss may reflect the impact of low levels of the vitamin in the gastrointestinal tract.

Cataracts can be related to low thiamine levels.

IS IT POSSIBLE TO GET TOO MUCH?
Because thiamine is a water-soluble vitamin, the body is very efficient at excreting excess in the urine. Therefore, there appear to be no adverse effects associated with high doses.

A day's Supereating

BREAKFAST
porridge sprinkled with wheat germ and sunflower seeds (all reasonable sources of magnesium); a teaspoon of blackstrap molasses will increase overall levels of B vitamins

LUNCH
stewed lentils with a mixed salad (gently stewing foods allows the nutrients that are water-soluble, such as B1, to be retained in the cooking liquid)

DINNER
pork loin cooked slowly with brown or red rice stuffing, steamed vegetables (slow cooking and steaming will not destroy or lose thiamine; wholegrain rice will contain most of the B vitamin family, while pork will provide B12)

Vitamin B2, also known as riboflavin, is another member of the water-soluble B vitamin family. Discovered as far back as 1879, it was identified as a B vitamin in 1933.

What are the best food sources?

The best food sources of riboflavin are dairy foods, particularly yoghurt, eggs and fish (particularly trout and tuna). Broccoli and spinach are the best green vegetable sources; avocados, red meat and dark chicken meat are also good sources. Grains are a good source, particularly oat bran, wheat germ, quinoa and rye.

How does the body use it?

Riboflavin is primarily recognized for its role in the formation of energy from glucose, protein and fats. It also plays an important part in the formation of thyroid hormone and works with iron to produce red blood cells. These functions make it a key player in maintaining energy levels. Because of its connection with iron, riboflavin has been used to treat some forms of anaemia.

Riboflavin is connected to several antioxidant reactions and is therefore protective against free radical damage. In this role, it has been shown to be protective against cataracts. It is also protective of the cardiovascular system, working with other B vitamins to reduce levels of a harmful substance called homocysteine (see Maintaining Heart Health, page 128).

Riboflavin has a particular connection with vitamin B3 (niacin) as it is needed to convert this family member from an amino acid called tryptophan.

Our immune response is partially dependent on riboflavin, as it helps us produce certain white blood cells.

Riboflavin can be effective in controlling migraines, although the exact process is still the subject of ongoing research.

✔ Friends

• **Other B vitamins** are needed for riboflavin pathways, particularly thiamine (but excess can have the opposite effect), folic acid and B6.
• Daily **live yoghurt** intake can increase levels of riboflavin.

✗ Foes

• **Low thyroid function and adrenal stress** can affect circulating levels of riboflavin.
• **Low levels of other B vitamins** can suppress riboflavin.
• **Excessive exercise** can increase demand.
• **Excessive alcohol consumption** suppresses riboflavin levels.
• Riboflavin is extremely sensitive to **light** (sunlight can lower riboflavin levels in milk by as much as 50%).

SEE ALSO

Other B vitamins, esp. B3 *pp32–47*   Probiotics *p86*   Boosting the Immune System *p106*
Eating for Greater Energy *p124*   Maintaining Heart Health *p128*   Maintaining General Skin Health *p136*

WHAT ARE THE SIGNS OF GETTING TOO LITTLE?
Signs of riboflavin deficiency typically include cracking and sores
in the corner of the mouth. Sore, watery and itching eyes could
also be symptoms, as could skin rash and peeling of the skin.

Because riboflavin is so important for energy production,
fatigue could be another symptom.

Pre-eclampsia, the high blood pressure that can occur
during pregnancy, is much more likely when levels of
riboflavin are low.

IS IT POSSIBLE TO GET TOO MUCH?
Like other B vitamins, riboflavin is easily
excreted, which makes it very difficult
to get too much. Just a word of
caution, though: high levels of
riboflavin can turn urine bright
yellow, which is quite
harmless but can be
rather startling.

A day's Supereating

BREAKFAST
*live yoghurt with oat bran and
soaked apricots (dried fruits contain
reasonable levels of riboflavin)*

LUNCH
*spinach omelette with a slice of rye
bread*

DINNER
*lamb stew, Moroccan-style with
apricots and pine nuts (pine nuts are
high in folic acid, while quinoa is a high-
riboflavin alternative to couscous)*

Vitamin B3,

also known as niacin, is another member of the vitamin B family. While the name 'niacin' refers to B3 generally, the vitamin actually exists in different chemical forms, which can be confusing. Nicotinic acid and nicotinamide (or sometimes niacinamide) all refer to forms of vitamin B3. These different names originated in the 1930s, when the vitamin was first isolated following research into the chemical nicotine, obtained from tobacco. Niacin is not only available from our food, we can also synthesize our own from the amino acid tryptophan. Like the other B vitamins, niacin is water-soluble and works closely with other members of the vitamin B family.

What are the best food sources?

High-protein foods, such as poultry, fish, red meat and liver, are the best sources of niacin. Chestnut mushrooms are also a very good source. Foods that are high in tryptophan will help boost niacin levels, so dairy foods and eggs would be good choices as are sweet potatoes, asparagus, dates and avocados.

Many cereals, breads, pastas and flours are enriched with niacin, but some of these may not be good nutritional choices.

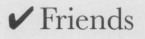

✔ Friends

• To form niacin from the amino acid tryptophan, the body requires **vitamins B2, B6 and iron.**
• **Other B vitamins** work with niacin. Low levels of B12 can lead to the loss of niacin in urine.
• Foods that are high in **tryptophan (dairy, eggs, poultry)** will help maintain niacin levels.

✗ Foes

• **Low-protein diets** may not provide sufficient tryptophan.
• **IBS and other digestive disorders** will significantly reduce absorption.
• Some drugs, such as **oral contraceptives**, can suppress niacin levels.
• **Heating** can release niacin from foods, so care may be needed with cooking methods.

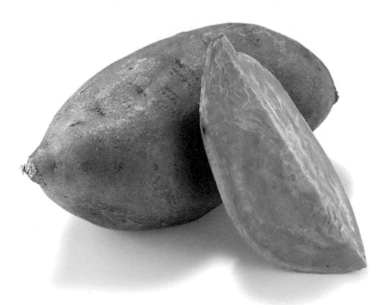

SEE ALSO

Other B Vitamins, esp. B2, B6 and B12 *pp32–47*   Iron *p58*   Improving Digestive Health *p118*   Eating for Greater Energy *p124*   Maintaining Heart Health *p128*   Maintaining General Skin Health *p136*

How does the body use it?

The main function of niacin is as an enzyme, facilitating important chemical reactions; in fact, it is involved in no less than 200 different enzymatic reactions. A well-recognized role of the vitamin is in the part it plays in the breakdown of carbohydrates, proteins and fats into energy. Niacin is therefore very important for maintaining energy levels, including energy production in the gastrointestinal (GI) tract, thus also making it important for effective digestion.

Niacin is also critical in the processing of fats and in the formation of the fatty acids needed in all cell membranes. Niacin is used in the liver for the production of cholesterol and there is plenty of research to show its importance for protecting our cardiovascular system and raising levels of HDL ('good') cholesterol.

Niacin appears to be involved in mechanisms controlling blood sugars, although research is ongoing to establish exactly how this works. There is, however, no disputing the protection it provides from some of the side effects of type-2 diabetes.

Niacin is also needed for healthy skin and has been shown to reduce the pain and inflammation caused by arthritis.

In view of its importance for the metabolizing of fat, it is not surprising that niacin is needed for healthy cells in the brain and nervous system. Research suggests that it is protective against cognitive decline.

Niacin also plays an important role in ensuring that our DNA is properly reproduced and can therefore play a role in the prevention and treatment of cancers.

WHAT ARE THE SIGNS OF GETTING TOO LITTLE?
Pellagra (with combined symptoms of weakness, diarrhoea, dementia and dermatitis) is the disease caused by major niacin deficiency and was the trigger for early research into this vitamin. This is a rare disease and is usually only a problem where corn is the staple diet.

Signs of niacin deficiency are general weakness and lack of appetite. Skin infections and irritation, as well as digestive problems, can also be related to low levels of niacin.

It is rare for Western diets to be low in niacin but if there is insufficient protein in the diet it could mean that levels of the amino acid tryptophan (from which the body makes its own niacin) are low, which could in turn result in low niacin.

IS IT POSSIBLE TO GET TOO MUCH?
Niacin is easily excreted in urine and there are no recorded incidences of toxicity resulting from the amounts provided by food.

Supplementing nicotinic acid at high levels can cause uncomfortable flushing and sweating.

A day's Supereating

BREAKFAST
poached egg, grilled chestnut mushrooms, whole grain toast (all good sources of niacin, tryptophan and riboflavin)

LUNCH
salad niçoise (tuna would provide niacin, riboflavin and B6; eggs would provide tryptophan)

DINNER
chicken braised with tomato and tomato paste, served with a leafy green vegetable such as broccoli and half a baked sweet potato (to provide tryptophan, B2, B6 and iron)

Vitamin B5, also known as pantothenic acid, is another member of the vitamin B family. Its name comes from the Greek word *pantos* meaning 'everywhere' as pantothenic acid is found throughout all living cells. In its active form, pantothenic acid is typically found as a substance called coenzyme A in plants, animals and food.

Water-soluble like all the members of the vitamin B family, pantothenic acid is readily absorbed right through the gastrointestinal (GI) tract. The beneficial bacteria in the colon make pantothenic acid, but it is not fully understood if this is used solely in the GI tract or if it adds to the total levels in the body and is used elsewhere as well.

✔ Friends

• **Biotin** works very closely with coenzyme A and is needed for many of its major functions.
• **Other members of the B vitamin family**, particularly folate and B12, are also needed for the chemical pathways involving pantothenic acid.
• There is evidence that **vitamin C** appears to prevent pantothenic deficiency.

✘ Foes

• Pantothenic acid in food is relatively unstable, so may be destroyed by **cooking**, **freezing** and **processing**.
• Digestion allows the release of coenzyme A from foods, so **impaired digestion** can reduce absorption.

What are the best food sources?

Pantothenic acid is found in all foods, but particularly good sources are liver and kidneys. Poultry and red meat are also good sources; dairy foods, particularly yoghurt, contain high levels and avocados are an excellent source. Of the pulses, lentils provide the highest levels. Tomato concentrate in paste and purée form provides good levels as well. Of the root vegetables, potatoes and sweet potato provide the best levels. Sunflower seeds also provide very high levels.

SEE ALSO

Vitamin C *p24*   Other B Vitamins, esp. Folic Acid and B12 *pp32–47*   Boosting the Immune System *p106*
Dealing with Stress *p112*   Maintaining Heart Health *p128*

How does the body use it?

As the name 'coenzyme A' suggests, the main function of pantothenic acid is enzymatic – it is involved in numerous chemical reactions throughout the body.

Its major function is in the generation of usable energy from carbohydrates, fats and proteins.

Pantothenic acid is also important for the synthesis of essential fats and other fat-related substances such as cholesterol and steroid hormones. These functions alone mean that it is present in the membrane of every cell in our body and is of particular importance to the nervous system. It not only forms part of the protective fatty covering of nerves, called the myelin sheath, but is also used to produce a particular neurotransmitter, one of the chemical messengers in the nervous system. Pantothenic acid also appears to play a role in improving cholesterol levels.

Vitamin B5 supports our adrenal glands and improves our response to stress. The importance of pantothenic acid in the formation of proteins makes it a key player in the many roles proteins play in our system, such as the transcribing of DNA and healthy cell division, the formation of antibodies and our immune responses, as well as the signalling mechanisms between cells.

Coenzyme A is needed for the synthesis of heme, an important component of our red blood cells. It is also needed for effective detoxification by the liver.

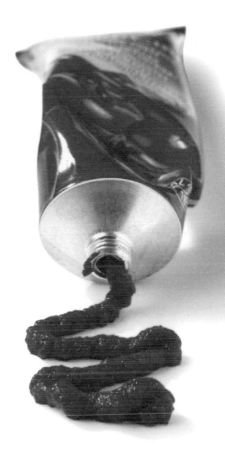

WHAT ARE THE SIGNS OF GETTING TOO LITTLE?
Deficiency is rare, but an imbalance could result in fatigue, poor handling of stress, and tingling or burning sensations in the feet.

IS IT POSSIBLE TO GET TOO MUCH?
There have been no incidences of pantothenic acid toxicity, with even controlled studies of mega-doses revealing no toxic effects.

A day's Supereating

BREAKFAST
plain yoghurt, fresh fruit, sunflower seeds, oat flakes (these will provide B5 and biotin as well as other B vitamins)

LUNCH
chicken and avocado salad (to provide pantothenic acid with other B vitamins)

DINNER
lamb shank braised with mushrooms and tomato paste, roast sweet potato (again this will provide pantothenic acid with a good range of other B vitamins)

Vitamin B6 is a general term covering a group of closely related compounds, the best known of which is pyridoxine. These are converted in the body into an active coenzyme, which in turn is used in over 100 different chemical reactions countless times every day. Like other family members it is water-soluble and its main activity is acting together with other enzymes to speed up chemical reactions. A notably hard-working member of the vitamin B family, vitamin B6 cannot be made in our bodies, therefore we need to obtain it entirely from our diet.

✔ Friends

- Vitamin B6 works closely with **other members of the B vitamin family, particularly folic acid and B12** in the conversion of homocysteine and riboflavin needed for red blood cell production.
- Effective metabolizing of **thiamine** is needed to maintain vitamin B6 function.

✘ Foes

- **Cooking and processing**, particularly freezing, lead to vitamin B6 loss from foods.
- **High levels of acid** during cooking can result in loss of vitamin B6.
- Some drugs, including the **contraceptive pill and diuretics**, can reduce B6 levels.

What are the best food sources?

Poultry, red meat and offal (particularly liver), as well as pulses (particularly chickpeas) and fish are all good sources of B6. Whole grains and brown rice provide good levels.

Green vegetables (particularly spinach) are good sources, as are asparagus, avocados, cauliflowers, sweet peppers and chestnut mushrooms. Root vegetables are also good sources, including carrots, sweet potatoes, leeks and onions.

Bananas and cantaloupe melon are the fruits providing the highest levels.

Cooking with turmeric and ginger could also improve levels.

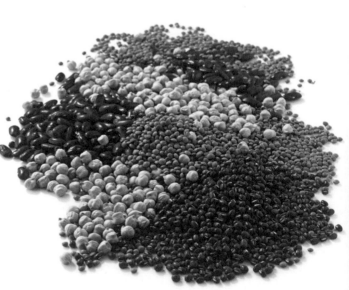

SEE ALSO

Other B Vitamins, esp. Folic Acid and B12 *pp32–47*   Magnesium *p60*   Boosting the Immune System *p106*
Dealing with Stress *p112*   Eating for Greater Energy *p124*   Maintaining General Skin Health *p136*

How does the body use it?

Vitamin B6 is particularly linked to the transformation and breakdown of proteins, giving it a key role in the formation of antibodies and our immune response, as well as in the formation of new cells.

B6 plays a big part in the different aspects of making energy: it is needed for the formation of red blood cells, which transport oxygen; it is needed for the release of glucose, and it is also needed for the use of protein for energy.

B6 is also important for the working of our nervous system, where it is used for the formation of different neurotransmitters, the chemical messengers that regulate our mood and mental processes. It is needed for the formation of tryptophan and can therefore help maintain niacin levels.

When first discovered, vitamin B6 was known as 'antidermatitis factor', which gives a clue to its importance in maintaining a healthy skin, due to its role in cell replication.

Working with folic acid and B12, B6 is one of the key nutrients needed in the metabolism of the amino acid homocysteine. The problems that this amino acid can cause when levels get too high include heart disease (see Maintaining Heart Health, page 128), poor cognitive function, osteoporosis, diabetes and problems with conception.

B6 can also modify the actions of our steroid hormones, which includes our sex hormones. This means it is possible that B6 could have a role in protection from some cancers, such as prostate and breast cancer. This action could also account for the relief B6 can give women suffering from the anxiety symptoms of premenstrual syndrome, when it works in conjunction with magnesium. B6 may also be helpful in alleviating the symptoms of morning sickness during pregnancy.

WHAT ARE THE SIGNS OF GETTING TOO LITTLE?
Mild deficiency appears to be quite common, with as many as 20% of women failing to meet the recommended target intake of 1–1.5mg daily.

Symptoms of mild deficiency would typically include irritability, depression and insomnia. A sore tongue, mouth ulcers and dermatitis are also signs.

Premenstrual syndrome symptoms can be related to low levels of vitamin B6.

Immune function, particularly in the elderly, can be impaired by low levels of vitamin B6.

IS IT POSSIBLE TO GET TOO MUCH?
In rare cases, prolonged doses of vitamin B6 at more than 200mg a day can cause nerve damage. More usually the toxic levels would need to be several times that limit.

A day's Supereating

BREAKFAST
porridge with yoghurt, ground flaxseeds and $1/2$ banana, sliced

LUNCH
chicken, avocado and sweet potato salad, with a ginger dressing

DINNER
veal escalope braised with mushrooms, leeks and onion on brown rice with turmeric

Note: all the above provide vitamin B6 in conjunction with other B vitamins

Biotin, occasionally referred to as vitamin B7 or vitamin H, is one of the less well-known of the B vitamins. It was discovered in the late 1930s, although it took much longer to establish that it was, in fact, a vitamin. It is water-soluble and can only be synthesized by bacteria, yeasts, moulds, algae and some plant species. While we obtain the majority of our biotin from food, it can also be synthesized by the bacteria in our gut, which produce small amounts themselves.

What are the best food sources?

Offal is a good source, particularly liver. Fish, egg yolk and soy products are excellent sources. Nuts, particularly hazelnuts and almonds, are good. Vegetables contain biotin, and Swiss chard, sweet potato, tomatoes, carrots and avocados all contain significant amounts.

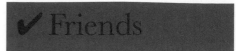

✔ Friends

- Healthy gut flora are needed to make our own biotin, so **probiotics** are friends.
- **B vitamins** work with biotin in many of its functions, but **vitamin B5** is particularly important.

✗ Foes

- **Disruption to gut bacteria balance** will affect our own production of biotin, so **antibiotics**, **Crohn's Disease and IBS** could all suppress levels.
- **Raw egg white** binds to biotin in the yolk, preventing absorption.
- Demand during **pregnancy** is much higher.
- **Food processing** can destroy biotin.
- **Strongly acidic conditions** in the digestive tract can destroy biotin.

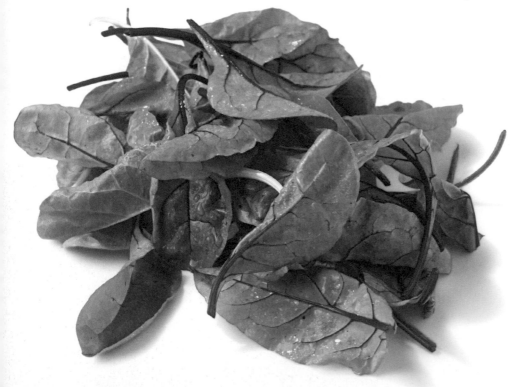

Other B Vitamins, esp. B5 *pp32–47*   **Probiotics** *p86*   **Dealing with Stress** *p112*
Eating for Greater Energy *p124*   **Maintaining Heart Health** *p128*

How does the body use it?

Like other B vitamins, biotin is used as an enzyme mainly working with other enzymes to speed up chemical reactions. Biotin works in particular with coenzyme A, the active form of vitamin B5, giving it a role in the formation of the essential fats that are the building blocks of every cell in the body. It is also involved in the processing of various proteins, and the formation of cholesterol (which is a necessary substance, and is only an issue when levels are considered too high).

Biotin is very important for producing energy from proteins and fats, as it is involved in the process of making energy in the cells.

Biotin plays an important role in maintaining blood sugar balance, not only through the processing of glucose but also because it is used in the formation of insulin.

Research into biotin is ongoing, and recent studies show that biotin plays a role in the formation of DNA and the control of cell replication. This would make it of particular importance in the prevention of cancer.

Because our nervous system uses both glucose and fat for energy, biotin is important for a healthy nervous system.

WHAT ARE THE SIGNS OF GETTING TOO LITTLE?

Biotin deficiency is very rare, but low levels typically show up in the skin and hair, with hair loss, a rash or red skin around the mouth, eyes and nose being possible signs. Cradle cap in infants and seborrheic dermatitis in adults are often related to low biotin levels. Brittle nails have also responded to increased biotin intake.

Depression and lethargy could also be signs, due to poor energy production and problems with the nervous system.

Low biotin could also be a reason for poor muscle tone and coordination, and muscle cramps.

IS IT POSSIBLE TO GET TOO MUCH?

Biotin is not known to be toxic, although long-term megadoses (several 1,000mg daily) of biotin and pantothenic acid (vitamin B5) taken together could be toxic.

A day's Supereating

BREAKFAST
mixed flake (oats and rice) porridge with soya milk, scattered with crushed nuts and $1/_2$ banana chopped (to provide biotin and B5 as well as other B vitamins)

LUNCH
grated carrot and sweet potato salad with hard-boiled egg and toasted almonds (to provide biotin with pantothenic acid and other B vitamins)

DINNER
white fish with mushrooms, Swiss chard and roasted sweet potato (again this will provide biotin with pantothenic acid and a good range of other B vitamins)

Folic Acid,

a member of the vitamin B family, is water-soluble and used throughout the body. It occurs in different forms, the best-known being as folates, the naturally occurring forms found in foods and the active forms found in our bodies. Folic acid is the most stable form of the vitamin and is the one most widely used in fortified foods and supplements.

Like other B vitamins, folic acid works closely with family members, particularly vitamins B6 and B12.

What are the best food sources?

As its names suggests, folic acid is found in green vegetables: Cos lettuce, avocado, asparagus, spinach and broccoli are the best. Better sources yet are pulses, particularly lentils. Liver provides the highest levels of folic acid.

Many cereals, breads, pastas and flours are enriched with folic acid, but some of these may not be good nutritional choices.

✔ Friends

• **Other members of the vitamin B family** (this includes thiamine, riboflavin, niacin, B6 and B12) are needed for many and varied biochemical processes.

✗ Foes

• **Problems with absorption,** such as **Crohn's or coeliac disease**, will result in low folic acid levels.
• **Low levels of vitamins B6 and B12** will suppress the action of folic acid.
• **High alcohol intake** is a risk factor for low folic acid.
• **Cooking and processing of vegetables** can destroy folic acid.
• **Pregnancy** significantly increases demand.

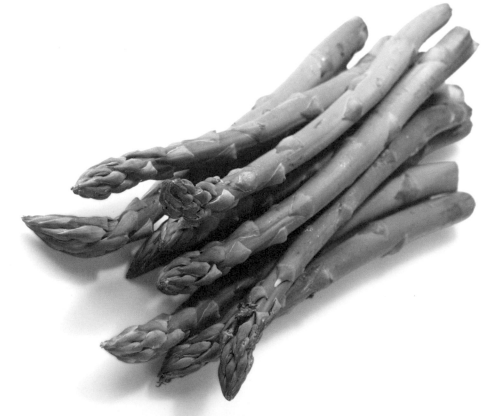

All B vitamins, especially B6 and B12 *pp32–47*   Zinc *p74*

How does the body use it?

Like other B vitamins, folic acid's main role is as an enzyme; i.e. a substance that converts compounds into a usable form. Its most critical function is in relation to DNA, which is effectively the 'blueprint' for every cell in our body. Folic acid is essential for the proper replication of our DNA, which gives it a leading role in healthy cell formation at the most basic level in every part of our body.

Folic acid is now widely recognized as being critical to the correct development of the neural tube in the foetus, which is the part where the baby's brain, spinal cord, spinal nerves and backbone will develop.

Folic acid works very closely with vitamins B6 and B12 in metabolizing the amino acid homocysteine. Research indicates that if the metabolism of this gets 'stuck', the resulting high levels in the system can lead to various conditions: heart disease is a well-documented risk of high levels of homocysteine (see Maintaining Heart Health, page 128); others include problems with conception, poor cognitive function, osteoporosis and even diabetes.

Because folic acid plays such an important role in the replication of cells it is not surprising that it can prevent cell mutation and cancer formation. Research suggests that cancers of the colon, breast and prostate can be linked to low folic acid levels.

Folic acid is also very closely connected with vitamin B6 in the formation of red blood cells.

WHAT ARE THE SIGNS OF GETTING TOO LITTLE?

One sign of severe folic acid deficiency is a certain kind of anaemia called megablastic anaemia. This relatively rare form occurs because the red blood cells are not correctly formed due to lack of folic acid, and is also linked to levels of vitamin B6.

A sore red tongue, chronic diarrhoea and poor growth in children are other signs of deficiency.

Cells that replicate quickly will be the first to show signs of folic acid deficiency, so gingivitis and periodontal disease may be linked to deficiency of this vitamin.

Birth defects can be a result of low folic acid.

Any risks related to high homocysteine would only show up in blood tests.

IS IT POSSIBLE TO GET TOO MUCH?

It is virtually impossible to get too much folate from foods, but mega-doses (over 5,000µg) in supplements may be dangerous for those with hormone-related cancers and epilepsy.

High levels of folic acid may inhibit zinc absorption.

A day's Supereating

BREAKFAST
poached egg on asparagus (to provide a mix of B vitamins as well as folic acid)

LUNCH
lentil salad with avocados (to provide a mix of B vitamins as well as folic acid)

DINNER
sautéed liver with mushrooms and a side salad of Cos lettuce, spinach and broccoli scattered with pine nuts (again this will provide folic acid with a good range of other B vitamins, particularly B12)

Vitamin B12, also known as cobalamin, is another

member of the vitamin B family. It was first discovered in 1934 but its chemical structure was not fully understood until the 1960s.

Unlike other nutrients, vitamin B12 is not actually made in animals or plants, unusually it originates from bacteria, fungi and algae. It is found in virtually all animal tissue and many – but by no means all – vegetables.

B12 is probably the most complicated of all the B vitamins, for several reasons. Firstly, it contains a mineral, cobalt, which makes it unique amongst the family of B vitamins – none of the others contain any mineral. Secondly, its method of absorption is far from straightforward and relies upon a combination of stomach acid, protein and a special carrier called 'intrinsic factor'.

Although water-soluble, like all the B family, B12 can be recycled and stored for many years and, while it is found throughout the body, we store the majority of it in our liver.

✔ Friends	✘ Foes
• **Other B vitamins** are needed for B12 enzymes, particularly riboflavin, folate and vitamin B6.	*Because of the different factors required for absorption, any missing step can result in deficiency:*

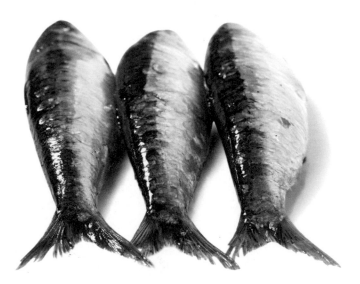

Foes (continued):

• **Anything that reduces stomach acid and gastric enzymes** can result in low B12 absorption. This can include medication such as antacids, stomach ulcers and old age.

• **Pernicious anaemia**, an autoimmune condition of the stomach that blocks the production of intrinsic factor.

• A **vegan diet** will have no obvious source of B12, although bacteria and fungi attached to fresh organic vegetables, particularly root vegetables, can provide B12.

• An **imbalance in other B vitamins** can suppress B12 pathways and high levels of folate can mask B12 deficiency.

Other B Vitamins, esp. B2, Folic Acid and B6 *pp32–47*   Boosting the Immune System *p106*
Dealing with Stress *p112*   Eating for Greater Energy *p124*   Maintaining Heart Health *p128*

How does the body use it?

Vitamin B12 in its various forms is used in two important enzymes, each having a range of functions.

The first enzyme is involved in the activation of proteins and particularly the synthesis of one amino acid, methionine. Through this action, B12 plays an active part in the appropriate replication of our DNA, which makes it important at a fundamental level for healthy cell formation. If cells do not replicate properly, these 'mutant' cells can become cancerous. Also through this enzyme B12 has a role in the formation of healthy sperm and in the control of homocysteine levels (a protein found in the blood that is linked to cardiovascular disease), where it works closely with B6 and folic acid. B12 is also important for maintaining the protective coating around our nerves and therefore a healthy nervous system.

The second enzyme is linked to the production of energy and the formation of haemoglobin and red blood cells, where it works together with other members of the B vitamin family.

B12 can also influence our sleep patterns, because it appears to influence the hormone melatonin, which is directly linked to inducing sleep.

WHAT ARE THE SIGNS OF GETTING TOO LITTLE?

Because we can store vitamin B12 for several years, deficiency takes time to develop.

Fatigue and anaemia can be signs of low levels of B12, due to poor energy production and problems with the formation of healthy red blood cells.

Nerve damage can be related to low vitamin B12 levels and signs can include numbness and tingling in our extremities, as well as memory loss, depression and dementia.

A sore red tongue and appetite loss can also be signs of B12 deficiency.

IS IT POSSIBLE TO GET TOO MUCH?

There have been no reported incidents of B12 toxicity, even when the vitamin has been injected in high doses. It is impossible to get toxic levels from food alone for two reasons: B12 is water-soluble and can easily be excreted, and the complicated absorption pathways make it hard to absorb very high levels.

What are the best food sources?

Animal-based foods are the best source of vitamin B12, with red meat, particularly liver, poultry and game, being good sources. Oily fish are high in B12. Eggs and dairy food contain B12, particularly fermented foods such as yoghurt.

A day's Supereating

BREAKFAST
poached egg on spinach with rye bread

LUNCH
wholegrain pasta salad with fresh tuna and green beans and a mixed salad

DINNER
casserole of chicken with mushrooms and tomatoes, steamed green vegetables

Note: all the above provide vitamin B12 in conjunction with other B vitamins

Boron is one of the minerals that is only required in trace, or very small, amounts. The true importance of boron did not become apparent to scientists until the mid-1980s and research into its functions is ongoing.

It is found in sea water and is therefore abundant in sea vegetables and fish, etc. Boron is also found in rocks and some soils, particularly in dry climates, and is accumulated in plants, although not necessarily used by them – they appear to be more a receptacle or carrier of the mineral. It appears that boron is easily leached from soils in wet climates.

Although it is not yet officially recognized as an 'essential' nutrient for human beings, data from recent research suggests that boron is important for a variety of functions and, in fact, may well be classed as an essential nutrient. The highest concentrations in the body are found in the bones.

What are the best food sources?

Nuts appear to provide the highest levels of boron, followed by fresh non-citrus fruits, like apples, avocados, raisins and tomatoes, and green vegetables, as well as pulses.

✔ Friends

• Boron appears to have an up-regulating effect on **vitamin D** – this makes it more of a friend for vitamin D.

✘ Foes

• More research needs to be carried out before we fully understand the mechanisms relating to the absorption and metabolism of boron and, consequently, any inhibitory factors.

SEE ALSO

Vitamin D *p26*   **Calcium** *p50*   **Magnesium** *p60*   **Improving Digestive Health** *p118*

How does the body use it?

Over the last fifteen years, intensive research has allowed us to understand the importance of boron, particularly for its role in strengthening bones and teeth, as it is involved in the metabolism of calcium and magnesium, as well as in enhancing cartilage formation. It is also recognized that boron plays an important role in the metabolism of steroid hormones, particularly testosterone and oestrogen, although the exact mechanisms of this are not yet understood. Other functions that are being investigated in relation to boron include those of the brain, particularly memory and concentration, as well as the absorption of dietary fat.

WHAT ARE THE SIGNS OF GETTING TOO LITTLE?

Due to its role in strengthening bone and cartilage formation, low bone density and osteoarthritis may be related to boron deficiency.

IS IT POSSIBLE TO GET TOO MUCH?

Boron toxicity is only likely through excessive supplementation – it is not recommended that any boron is supplemented during pregnancy or breastfeeding.

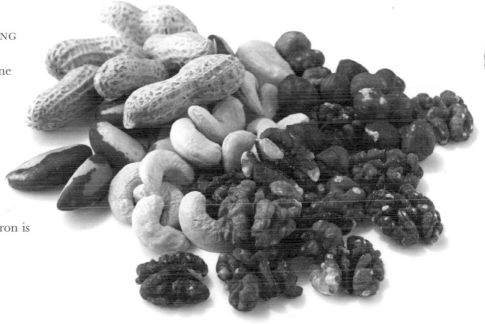

A day's Supereating

BREAKFAST
live yoghurt with chopped apples and pears, muesli with mixed nuts

LUNCH
avocado salad tossed with broad beans

DINNER
mixed bean stew with stir-fried carrot and cabbage sprinkled with lightly toasted crushed nuts

Note: remember also to drink at least 1.5 litres of water during the day – this will provide additional boron

Calcium, along with vitamin C, are perhaps among the best-known nutrients. Most of us become aware of the need for calcium from quite a young age, as it is so closely linked with bone health and is also promoted through milk intake for youngsters.

Calcium is known as a 'macro-mineral', indicating that we have more than 5g in the body and we need another 900mg a day from food or other sources, although the recommended intake is dependent on age and gender, and increases considerably during breast-feeding. Calcium is the most prolific mineral found in the human body. About 99% of the body's calcium is stored in our bones; the remainder is found circulating in the blood and in the fluid around our cells.

✔ Friends

- **Vitamin D** (mainly produced in the skin when it is exposed to sunlight, but also available from oily fish) is essential for calcium absorption and metabolism.
- **Magnesium** (found in most foods, including fish, grains, green leafy vegetables, seeds and dairy foods) works synergistically with calcium, and an imbalance of one can affect the absorption and metabolism of the other. Research shows that the ideal ratio between the two minerals, in most circumstances, is 2 parts magnesium to 1 part calcium.
- **Potassium** (found mainly in fruit and vegetables) appears to reduce calcium excretion in the urine.
- **Inulin** (the soluble fibre found in fruits and vegetables such as asparagus, garlic and Jerusalem artichokes) can increase calcium absorption in the colon.
- **Probiotics** appear to increase the absorption of calcium from dairy foods (as found in yoghurt and cottage cheese).
- The **essential fatty acids** may help the absorption of calcium.

✘ Foes

The following can prevent the absorption of calcium from food:
- **Phytates**, found in bran, legumes, some nuts and seeds.
- **Oxalates**, found in spinach, some soft fruits, quinoa, almonds and peanuts.
- **Low hydrochloric acid** in the stomach, which can result from stress or poor zinc status.
- **Tannins** found in tea and coffee.

The following can increase the demand for calcium:
- **Refined sugar.**
- **Phosphoric acid**, found mainly in fizzy drinks.
- **High-protein diets.**

The following can upset calcium metabolism
- **Coffee** interferes with factors that regulate calcium metabolism, such as inositol.
- **Salt** can increase calcium excretion in the urine.

SEE ALSO

Vitamin D *p26*   Magnesium *p60*   Potassium *p66*   Probiotics *p86*   EFAs *p90*   Maintaining Heart Health *p128*

How does the body use it?

Calcium is widely recognized for its role in bone health, providing both strength and structure to bones and teeth. However, it also plays other very important roles that are not so widely known, such as being utilized by cells for communicating with one another. This includes involvement in the constriction and relaxation of blood vessels and the transmission of nerve impulses, the contraction and relaxation of muscles, and the secretion of some hormones such as insulin. Bear in mind that the heart is a large muscle that expands and contracts about 100–150 times a minute, so calcium has a major role in heart health.

Calcium is also very important for blood clotting, because it is used to activate the different clotting factors and so wound healing and recovery are partially dependent on adequate calcium levels.

Calcium and vitamin D together may also play a role in preventing breast cancer.

WHAT ARE THE SIGNS OF GETTING TOO LITTLE?

Because the majority of calcium is stored in bones, when calcium intake is low the body compensates by borrowing from these stores to carry out any of the above functions, resulting in poor bone density – which can then lead to osteoporosis.

Other deficiency signs include muscle cramps and hypertension or increased blood pressure.

IS IT POSSIBLE TO GET TOO MUCH?

Over-high levels of calcium can occur from food sources, but only extremely rarely. It is more common in someone consuming excess calcium-containing medication, such as antacids, combined with supplements and milk. This would result in a condition called hypercalcaemia, with effects such as lethargy, headaches and confusion.

What are the best food sources?

The best natural food sources of calcium are soft fish bones, so eat plenty of whitebait and sardines. Tinned salmon, with its soft bones, is also excellent. These food sources have the advantage of also being natural sources of vitamin D, which will further enhance calcium absorption.

Good vegetarian sources are fermented dairy products, such as plain live yoghurt and cottage cheese. Soya yoghurt and tofu that have been fortified both supply easily absorbable calcium. Cheddar cheese is high in calcium, but its high saturated fat content means it should be eaten only in moderation.

There are good levels of calcium in Chinese lettuce and reasonable levels in pak choy, kale, broccoli, pulses, soya beans, almonds and sesame seeds.

Remember, if you are in a hard water area, tap water will be high in calcium carbonate.

A day's Supereating

BREAKFAST
live yoghurt with sesame seeds, oats and soaked prunes (to provide calcium from a probiotic source and magnesium)

LUNCH
smoked mackerel with a mixed salad to include watercress, broccoli florets and asparagus, scattered with sesame and sunflower seeds (to provide calcium, inulin, magnesium and vitamin D)

DINNER
stir-fried pak choy with garlic and ginger, sprinkled with toasted almonds, served with freshly grilled sardines and lemon juice; a vegetarian choice could include marinated tofu rather than sardines (to provide calcium, magnesium and vitamin D)

Chromium is a familiar

metal, but more research is needed to establish the full extent of its different roles in the body. Our stores of chromium are found mainly in the skin, body fat, adrenal glands, muscle tissue and the brain, and are transported around the body in two forms, the most common being Glucose Tolerance Factor (GTF) which is made from chromium combined with vitamin B3 and glutathione.

Chromium is recognized as an essential nutrient but is needed only in trace (very small) amounts. The lack of information on this mineral means that there is no recommended daily intake, but general scientific opinion suggests that an adequate daily intake is 50μg. However, daily intakes of 200μg have been shown to be safe and higher levels could be indicated in cases of deficiency, although taking high levels without proper supervision and monitoring is not advised.

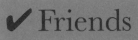

✔ Friends

• Adequate levels of **vitamin B3 and glutathione** are needed to make the active form of chromium, GTF.
• **Vitamin C** increases absorption.

✗ Foes

• A diet of **refined food, high in sugar and carbohydrates** increases the demand for chromium.
• **Trauma and mental stress** increase chromium excretion.
• **Calcium carbonate** (mainly found in hard water) and **phytic acid** (found in coffee, whole grains and legumes) both decrease absorption of chromium.

SEE ALSO

Vitamin C *p24*   Vitamin B3 *p36*   Improving Digestive Health *p118*
Eating for Greater Energy *p124*   Maintaining Heart Health *p128*

How does the body use it?

It is now understood that the primary role of chromium is in the management of glucose. It facilitates the uptake of glucose into cells by strengthening the binding properties of the glucose storage hormone insulin. It is therefore a key nutrient for handling insulin resistance and type-2 diabetes, and can be helpful for weight loss, although it is no magic bullet.

Due to its ability to improve the effectiveness of insulin, chromium also appears to play a role in breaking down protein and fat, although more research needs to be done. There is evidence that chromium helps to reduce plaque formation on blood vessels, suggesting that it can be beneficial in the prevention of heart attacks and strokes.

WHAT ARE THE SIGNS OF GETTING TOO LITTLE?
High blood sugar levels are the primary sign of chromium deficiency, combined with the symptoms of insulin resistance, such as fatigue, weight gain, pre-menstrual syndrome.

Other deficiency signs include low levels of HDL ('good' cholesterol) and high blood pressure.

IS IT POSSIBLE TO GET TOO MUCH?
It is not possible to get toxic levels of chromium from food, but excess chromium is toxic and can result in anaemia and liver damage. However, this would need levels in excess of ten times the maximum limits found in supplements.

What are the best food sources?

Chromium is not widely available in staple foods. Good food sources include raw onion, tomato, black pepper, liver, poultry, shellfish, broccoli, brewer's yeast, whole grains, pulses, spices and grape juice.

A day's Supereating

BREAKFAST
unsweetened red grape juice, whole grain muesli with wheat germ, nuts, yoghurt

LUNCH
prawn salad with rye bread
(this would provide niacin as well as chromium)

DINNER
sautéed liver with green peppers and mushrooms, stir-fried cabbage; a good vegetarian choice would be to make a frittata with the peppers and mushrooms (this would provide chromium along with niacin)

Copper is an essential mineral
that we need in trace (very small) amounts. At approximately 75mg, it is the third most abundant essential trace mineral in the human body and is distributed among all our organs, the highest concentrations being found in the brain and liver. Perhaps our most common experience of copper is the metal bands that many people with arthritis wear on the wrists, as it has been shown to reduce joint pain and inflammation.

✔ Friends

• **Selenium** and copper are both involved in numerous enzyme reactions.

✗ Foes

• High levels of **manganese, iron, zinc** and **vitamin C** have been shown to induce copper deficiency.
• **Phosphorus** and **calcium** in high levels can encourage copper excretion.
• The **contraceptive pill** can result in over-high copper levels.
• The consumption of high levels of **fructose** (fruit sugars) can result in copper deficiency.
• **Low levels of stomach acid.**

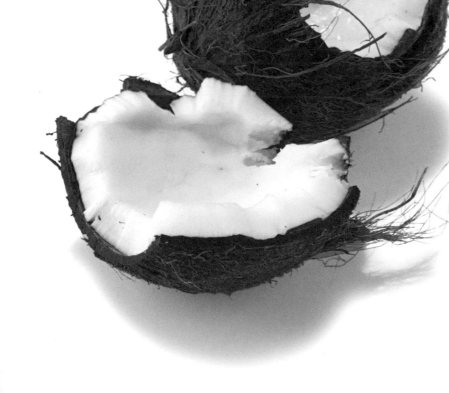

SEE ALSO

Vitamin C *p24*   Calcium *p50*   Iron *p58*   Manganese *p62*   Phosphorus *p64*
Selenium *p68*   Zinc *p74*   Eating for Greater Energy *p124*   Maintaining General Skin Health *p136*

How does the body use it?

As early as 400BC Hippocrates is said to have used copper to treat diseases, though we are still learning more about how and where it is used.

The most widespread use of copper is as a vital component of a large number of essential enzymes. As such it has two important roles in the formation of energy: it is involved both in the transport of iron to form red blood cells and in the metabolism of glucose into energy. Its other enzymatic functions involve the central nervous system, particularly brain function, as well as the pigmentation of hair, skin and eyes. Copper is also required for effective thyroid function and the formation of collagen.

Another very important function of copper is as an antioxidant, which helps protect the body from the damage caused by free radicals.

WHAT ARE THE SIGNS OF GETTING TOO LITTLE?
Copper deficiency is relatively uncommon, but anaemia that is unresponsive to iron therapy can respond to copper supplementation. Raised cholesterol (particularly 'bad' LDL), hair loss, weight gain, compromised immunity and depression could all be signs of reduced copper levels. Osteoporosis, joint pain and skin sores may all be related to copper deficiency because of its importance in the formation of collagen.

IS IT POSSIBLE TO GET TOO MUCH?
Eating foods that contain copper should provide more than adequate levels. Supplementation is rarely required, especially when you consider that levels of 900µg are considered the maximum for an adult.

What are the best food sources?

Copper is widely distributed in different foods, but good sources include shellfish, offal, miso, sesame and sunflower seeds, coconut milk, cashews, avocados, asparagus, garlic, chestnut mushrooms, beans, soya beans and oat bran.

A day's Supereating

BREAKFAST
porridge with live yoghurt, oat bran, sunflower seeds and blackberries

LUNCH
mixed bean salad with avocado, sprinkled with toasted soya nuts

DINNER
pan-fried calves' liver with asparagus; a vegetarian choice would be marinated tofu and sprouted mung beans stir-fried with coconut milk and cashews

Iodine is an essential mineral that is needed in trace, or very small, amounts. Unlike most minerals it is not metallic, and is found mainly in sea water and sea vegetables, such as kelp. Iodine is also found in certain soils, although erosion can leach it from the soil and many areas in the world are severely iodine deficient.

The body stores about 17mg of iodine, which is mainly found in the thyroid gland, but is also found in the stomach lining, salivary glands and in the blood as well.

What are the best food sources?

The best food sources of iodine are seafoods, saltwater fish and sea vegetables. Other vegetable sources depend on the iodine content of the soil on which they were grown. Dairy foods can be a good source of iodine when the cattle feed has been supplemented. Many herds of cattle are reared on feed that has been supplemented with nutrients, including iodine. This is often not specified when buying dairy produce from shops but if you buy directly from the farm then do ask.

✔ Friends

• **Selenium** can support thyroid function even when iodine is deficient.
• **Iron** and **vitamin A** are needed for iodine metabolism in relation to thyroid function.

✘ Foes

There are several foods that have been termed 'goitrogenic', which basically means they block the uptake of iodine, inducing deficiency. These are generally not of major clinical importance unless they form a major part of the diet in iodine-deficient areas. However, eaten in high quantities they can suppress thyroid function. Goitrogenic foods include:

- **Soya-based foods**
- **Raw cruciferous vegetables** (broccoli, cabbage etc.)
- **Red rice**
- **Millet**
- **Cassava**

How does the body use it?

Iodine is probably best known for its role in the production of thyroid hormones and, as such, it is important for metabolic regulation. When the thyroid output is impaired, the gland can expand like a sponge in an effort to try to grab more iodine from the blood, and this can lead to a swelling, or goitre, at the base of the throat, which is a common physical indication of low thyroid action.

Thyroid hormones regulate the development of the brain during pregnancy and during breast feeding, and therefore sufficient iodine is vital at these stages of our development.

WHAT ARE THE SIGNS OF GETTING TOO LITTLE?
Iodine deficiency is fairly common throughout the world, particularly in parts of India, Bangladesh and Burma, where iodine levels in the soils are very low. Even here, low iodine levels have also been identified in parts of Derbyshire.

Goitre formation on the neck is a familiar sign of severe iodine deficiency.

Earlier deficiency signs include fatigue, weight gain and reduced body temperature.

Miscarriage can be induced by low iodine and deficiency during pregnancy can lead to abnormal foetal brain development and cretinism.

IS IT POSSIBLE TO GET TOO MUCH?
Iodine toxicity is rare, but symptoms include raised heart rate and swollen throat. Watch intake from supplements in addition to food.

A day's Supereating

BREAKFAST
oat porridge with whole milk and topped with cashew nuts

LUNCH
smoked haddock chowder with wakame or other dried sea vegetables crushed into it

DINNER
seafood stir-fry

Iron is a very familiar and well-researched essential nutrient that is found in every cell of the human body. The general belief concerning iron is that it is found only in red meat, which is not the case.

Iron is a mineral that can be stored by the body and it normally contains between 3.5g and 4.5g. The majority of this iron, about 60%, is carried in the red blood cells. The remainder is found mainly in the liver, spleen, bone marrow and muscles.

Dietary iron is available in two distinct forms: 'heme' iron, which is found only in animal flesh, and 'non-heme' iron, which is found in plant foods and dairy products. Research suggests that heme iron is more absorbable than non-heme iron, although the overall amount of iron absorbed is also regulated by the body's need for iron. The recommended daily intake for iron is 8.7mg for men and post-menopausal women, and 14.8mg a day for young women.

✔ Friends

The following enhance absorption:

- **Amino acid intake**, particularly of cysteine (poultry, yoghurt, egg yolks, garlic, onions, oats, wheat germ, Brussels sprouts and broccoli are all good sources of cysteine).
- **Lactic acid** (found in fermented foods such as yoghurt, sourdough bread, sauerkraut, pickled cucumber, olives and kefir).
- **Citric acid** (citrus fruits, pineapple).
- **Tartaric acid** (found in grapes and grape juice products).
- **Malic acid** (sour apples, under-ripe fruit, tomatoes).
- **Ascorbic acid** (vitamin C).
- **Probiotics.**
- **Vitamin A** is required for effective iron metabolism.
- **Copper** is required for iron transport and iron storage.
- **Calcium** can bind to oxalic and phytic acid, thereby facilitating iron absorption.

✘ Foes

The following can reduce absorption of iron:

- **Tannins**, found in tea, coffee, chocolate, apple juice, red wine, beans, nuts, cigarette smoke and many fruits.
- **Polyphenols**, found in red wine, chocolate, legumes, many fruits and vegetables, many grains.
- **Phosphoric acid**, found mainly in fizzy drinks, beer and ice cream.
- The food additive **EDTA**.
- **Phytic acid and oxalic acid** can affect iron absorption by binding to the mineral.
- **Zinc** supplementation and high levels of **calcium** intake (including calcium phosphate found in baking powders, toothpaste and some supplements), probably because they compete for the same binding sites.
- **Low stomach acid** (particularly due to use of antacids).

SEE ALSO
- -

Vitamin A *p22*   Vitamin C *p24*   Calcium *p50*   Copper *p54*   Zinc *p74*
Boosting the Immune System *p106*   Eating for Greater Energy *p124*

How does the body use it?

The most familiar use for iron is in the delivery of oxygen in the blood from the lungs to cells, via haemoglobin; it also transports and stores oxygen within muscle cells, via myoglobin, providing them with a constant supply of oxygen to meet their demands. In addition, iron acts as an enzyme in the metabolic pathways that turn glucose into energy. This explains why iron is such a vital nutrient for energy production in every cell of the body.

Iron is also important for our immune defence system, because it forms part of several antioxidant enzymes, triggering reactions that protect cells from free radical damage.

WHAT ARE THE SIGNS OF GETTING TOO LITTLE?
Because iron plays such an important role in energy production, the first signs of deficiency are usually related to fatigue and include breathlessness and dizziness. Other signs can include brittle nails, a sore tongue and cracks at the side of the mouth, as well as pale skin, gums and nails. Iron deficiency signals often appear well before clinical signs of anaemia, which show up in a blood test as a low red blood cell count and low haemoglobin levels.

The primary cause for low iron is heavy blood loss, which could be due to trauma, menstruation or gastro-intestinal bleeding, as well as increased blood volume as in pregnancy.

IS IT POSSIBLE TO GET TOO MUCH?
It is possible to get too much iron, although this is generally via supplementation and highly unlikely with food. A hereditary condition, haemochromatosis, leads to high iron levels and is routinely tested for if iron levels are elevated.

What are the best food sources?

Good sources of iron include liver, beef, lamb and venison. Good vegetarian sources include chickpeas, beans and peas, chard and spinach, dried apricots, tomato paste, curry powder and ginger.

A day's Supereating

BREAKFAST
glass of freshly squeezed orange juice, live yoghurt with soaked dried apricots and a generous tablespoon of toasted oat flakes

LUNCH
stewed chickpeas cooked with onions, tomatoes, tomato paste, garlic and a squeeze of lemon juice

DINNER
venison liver sautéed with onions, orange juice and garlic, broccoli and peas; for a vegetarian option, sauté onions and orange juice with shredded garlic and top with a poached egg, serving with broccoli and peas as before

Magnesium

is perhaps the most prolific mineral in the body after calcium. Although we store less than 30g of this mineral, it is vital to hundreds of metabolic functions. 60% of our body stores are found in the bones and 25% in muscle cells, but only 1% is found in fluids outside cells.

✔ Friends

• Adequate **calcium** intake is needed for magnesium balance.
• It appears that **vitamin D** can help increase magnesium absorption but magnesium is not dependent on vitamin D in the same way as calcium.

✘ Foes

• **Phosphoric acid**, found mainly in sweet fizzy drinks, increases the demand for magnesium.
• **Oxalic acid** can inhibit magnesium absorption.
• **Insufficient calcium** intake appears to disrupt magnesium balance.
• **Highly processed grains** will be depleted of magnesium.

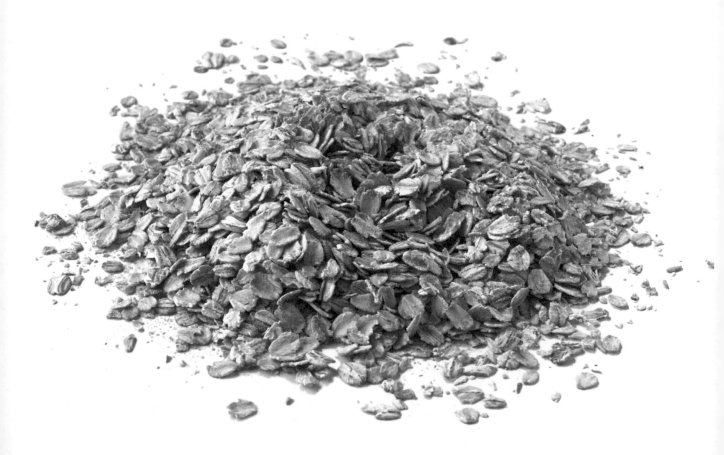

Vitamin D *p26*   Calcium *p50*   Dealing with Stress *p112*   Eating for Greater Energy *p124*

How does the body use it?

Magnesium is a truly versatile nutrient and plays an important role in a wide variety of functions. It works closely – and has an affinity – with calcium in providing the structural 'bone scaffolding' into which calcium and other minerals can slot; it also plays a role in the structural formation of cell membranes and chromosomes.

Magnesium is widely recognized as an 'anti-stress' mineral, due to its involvement in ion transportation, which affects muscle contraction, nerve impulse and normal heart rhythm. These functions account for its use in easing menstrual cramps and in treating asthma and bronchitis. It also helps the functioning of the adrenal glands and so is involved with adrenaline production, a further link to the factors that dictate how we handle stress.

Magnesium is not widely recognized for other important roles that do, however, deserve a mention. These include blood clotting, cell signalling, the synthesis of DNA, the formation of important enzymes involved in carbohydrate and lipid metabolism and the production and use of insulin.

Magnesium's starring role, however, is in energy production, where many of the chemical reactions needed to turn a molecule of glucose into ATP (which is the useable form of energy created by cells, see Eating for Greater Energy, p124) are dependent on magnesium.

WHAT ARE THE SIGNS OF GETTING TOO LITTLE?
Many of the signs of magnesium deficiency relate to its function as an 'anti-stress' mineral. So, insomnia, muscle cramps, twitching, increased heart rate and high blood pressure are all common symptoms of low magnesium levels. Muscle weakness, high blood fats, constipation and imbalanced blood glucose levels are other common signs of magnesium deficiency.

IS IT POSSIBLE TO GET TOO MUCH?
There is no evidence that we can get too much magnesium from food but, as with most minerals, supplementing magnesium can lead to excess. This often results in diarrhoea.

What are the best food sources?

Excellent food sources of magnesium include oat bran, brown rice, quinoa, pumpkin and sunflower seeds, whole grains, nuts, lentils and dark green leafy vegetables – which means that vegetarians will find it easy to obtain optimum levels of this important mineral.

Water can also be a source of magnesium, although levels vary between sources (tap and branded bottled water).

A day's Supereating

BREAKFAST
live yoghurt, porridge with added bran, mixed seeds

LUNCH
brown rice and lentil salad, with green leaves

DINNER
stir-fried prawns in coconut milk, quinoa and stir-fried shredded cabbage, spinach and pak choy

Manganese is a trace

mineral that is essential, although it is also potentially toxic, but not from ingesting it. Like so many of the trace minerals, more research is needed to understand fully its functions and mechanisms in the body. Appropriately, therefore, its name is derived from the Greek word for magic.

Manganese occurs naturally in many types of rock and in water. Manganese can also be combined with carbon to make pesticides and fuel additives.

✔ Friends

No research exists to highlight any friends of this mineral.

✘ Foes

The following may prevent the absorption of manganese from food:
- **Phytates** (found in coffee, whole grains, legumes).
- **Oxalates** (found in spinach and rhubarb in high levels).
- The **birth control pill** may depress manganese levels.
- Manganese levels depend on effective bile production, so an **overworked liver due to high alcohol intake** can suppress manganese.
- **Excessive supplementation of other minerals, such as zinc, magnesium, copper, iron and calcium** may suppress manganese levels.
- **Heavy sweating** may result in excessive loss of manganese.

Vitamin C *p24*   Vitamin B1 *p32*   Biotin *p42*   **Eating for Greater Energy** *p124*

How does the body use it?

Manganese is involved in the formation of a variety of enzymes and, as such, plays a role in many different metabolic functions. It is very important in the formation of the antioxidant responsible for protecting cells from the collateral damage of burning oxygen for energy (known as oxidative stress). It also plays an important part in maintaining healthy bones and in the metabolism of glucose and fat into energy. Manganese is required for effective wound healing, for the maintenance of healthy cholesterol levels and is involved in the metabolism of proteins. It is also important for memory and cognitive function.

Manganese also helps your body utilize key nutrients such as vitamin C, biotin and thiamine (vitamin B1).

WHAT ARE THE SIGNS OF GETTING TOO LITTLE?

Manganese deficiency is very rare in humans and usually does not develop unless manganese is deliberately eliminated from the diet. Because manganese is involved in so many enzymatic functions, deficiency may result in a wide variety of symptoms: poor blood sugar handling and the condition know as metabolic syndrome, skeletal deformity, low cholesterol levels, skin rash, dermatitis and vomiting, and even convulsions. Low manganese levels can impair growth and reproductive function.

IS IT POSSIBLE TO GET TOO MUCH?

Manganese is not easily absorbed from food, so it is not possible to get toxic levels just from food or even supplements. The only recorded cases of toxicity involve prolonged exposure to the mineral during mining and smelting. Low iron levels and poor liver clearance can increase the risk of excess manganese in the body.

What are the best food sources?

The best natural food sources of manganese are pineapple, nuts (particularly pecans, pine nuts, soya nuts and almonds), whole grains (particularly oats and oat bran), brown rice, beans, chickpeas, sweet potato, green leafy vegetables such as spinach, cinnamon, cloves and thyme.

Manganese is not found in any useful amounts in meat or dairy products.

A day's Supereating

BREAKFAST

pineapple chunks scattered with crushed almonds, followed by porridge made with water, plus additional oat bran and a pinch of ground cloves and cinnamon

LUNCH

baked sweet potato and cottage cheese with garlic and pine nuts

DINNER

chickpeas stewed with onion, garlic, tomatoes and thyme, scattered with lightly toasted soya nuts, stir-fried green cabbage or kale with garlic

Phosphorus

Phosphorus is a 'macro-mineral' that is used throughout the body, where it is second only to calcium in quantity. It is therefore not surprising to find that approximately 85% of this essential mineral is found stored in our bones, the remainder mainly being found in cell membranes. The recommended daily intake for phosphorus is 500mg.

Phosphorus is found plentifully in all living forms and in nature, as in our bodies, it is not found as a pure mineral but it is usually linked to oxygen to form a phosphate (which is a salt of phosphoric acid).

What are the best food sources?

Most foods contain phosphorus, so whether omnivore or vegetarian there is no problem obtaining sufficient phosphorus from the diet.

Good sources include seafoods, particularly roes, meat, particularly liver, eggs and dairy foods, pulses, quinoa, nuts and seeds.

✔ Friends

• **Vitamin D and calcium** are both needed for effective phosphorus utilization in bone formation.

✗ Foes

• High dietary intake of **fructose** (fruit sugars), particularly when combined with a **low intake of magnesium**, has been shown to increase the excretion of phosphorus.

• **Aluminium-containing antacids** reduce the absorption of dietary phosphorus.

Vitamin D *p26*   Calcium *p50*   Dealing with Stress *p112*   Improving Digestive Health *p118*
Maintaining General Skin Health *p136*

How does the body use it?

Phosphorus is a fascinating mineral that has many and varied functions in our body. It is mainly used in bone structure, where it combines with calcium to produce a very hard salt called hydroxyapatite. It is also used in the formation of collagen and tendons, so has two important roles in a healthy skeletal system. Collagen is part of all connective tissue, so phosphorus is also important for healthy eyes and skin.

Phosphorus plays several vital roles in fat handling. For example, our cell membranes use phosphorus in a very interesting way, by linking phosphorus with fats to form phospholipids, which allows the membranes to become soluble in both water and fat. This means that all nutrients, whether water- or fat-soluble can pass in or out of our cells. Phospholipids also act as a sort of detergent on fats in the blood, keeping the molecules small and the blood more fluid; they also help to break down digested fats and stop fats accumulating in the liver.

Phosphorus is also a major player in our nervous system: it makes up about one-third of the dry weight of our brain, forms part of the fatty sheath that protects our nerves and is vital as a cell-to-cell messenger.

In addition, phosphorus is the main component of our primary source of energy (ATP); so muscles not only need phosphorus to receive the nervous message to contract, they also need it to give them the energy to do so.

WHAT ARE SIGNS OF GETTING TOO LITTLE?
Because phosphorus is found so widely in all foods, deficiency is extremely rare and would require severe starvation. The primary deficiency signs naturally involve bone formation, so bone pain, rickets and osteomalacia could be signs, as could muscle weakness, tingling in the extremities and difficulty in walking as well as poor nervous function, poor cognitive function and loss of concentration.

IS IT POSSIBLE TO GET TOO MUCH?
It is more likely that one would see signs of excess phosphorus in a Western diet than in others. Most processed foods contain high levels of phosphorus in the form of polyphosphate food additives, while carbonated drinks in particular are high in phosphoric acid. High phosphorus levels may lead to calcium loss and low vitamin D formation.

A day's Supereating

BREAKFAST
scrambled egg scattered with ground pumpkin seeds

LUNCH
fish chowder or lentil soup

DINNER
sautéed liver with quinoa or oyster mushrooms and chestnut mushroom quinoa 'risotto'

Note: all the above will provide good levels of phosphorus with additional calcium

Potassium

is an essential mineral and the fourth most abundant mineral in the human body. 98% of it is found inside cells and these concentrations need to be tightly regulated for all normal body functions. Reserves of potassium are held in the liver and the muscles.

While the adult reference nutrient intake for potassium is 3,500mg, it appears that many people get less than 2,500mg daily, which is not ideal. Potassium is easily excreted in urine.

What are the best food sources?

Vegetables and fruit are the best sources of potassium and, because potassium is so easily excreted, these need to be eaten regularly – the 'five-a-day' rule is really important for potassium.

Potatoes are particularly high in potassium, but better still are avocados, tomato paste, sun-dried tomatoes and dried fruit. Squash, sweet potatoes, cucumbers, peppers, tomatoes, bananas and apricots are all good sources, and dark green vegetables are also excellent.

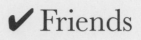

✔ Friends

No research exists to highlight any friends of this mineral.

✗ Foes

The modern Western diet is often potassium-suppressant because the high salt content upsets the delicate sodium/potassium balance in cells.

The main reasons for low potassium are linked to potassium loss and there are various causes for this:

• Long-term use of **diuretics** can cause potassium excretion in the urine.
• **Diarrhoea** is a very common cause for short-term potassium loss but **overuse of laxatives** could encourage long-term excretion.
• Potassium can be lost in sweat, so **over-exercising and extreme heat** can decrease potassium levels.
• Long-term **licorice** ingestion, through teas and supplements, can increase potassium excretion.

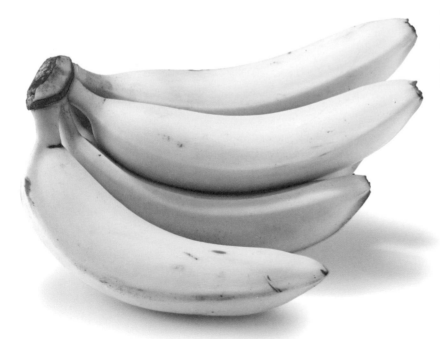

Sodium *p70*   **Eating for Greater Energy** *p124*   **Maintaining Heart Health** *p128*

How does the body use it?

The most important function of potassium is as an electrolyte; that is, a substance capable of conducting electricity when in a solution. In this form it performs a host of vital functions, in particular conducting nerve impulses for muscle contractions and regulating heartbeat.

Potassium works with sodium to maintain fluid levels inside and outside of cell membranes. This action makes it important for fluid excretion and retention, which therefore means it plays a role in reducing high blood pressure.

Potassium is also needed for the metabolism of proteins, as well as to activate certain enzymes, particularly in the formation of energy from glucose.

WHAT ARE THE SIGNS OF GETTING TOO LITTLE?

Although acute potassium deficiency is extremely rare, low levels can induce muscle weakness and headaches as well as arrhythmia and irritability. Water retention and consequent high blood pressure are also deficiency signals, because low potassium induces sodium retention.

IS IT POSSIBLE TO GET TOO MUCH?

There are no reported cases of toxicity from food sources because potassium is easily excreted in urine. However, there have been cases of cardiac arrest from ingesting high doses of potassium salt substitutes.

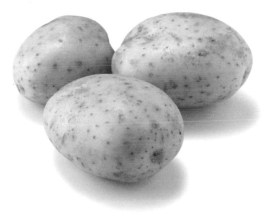

A day's Supereating

BREAKFAST
plain yoghurt, dried unsulphured apricots, soaked overnight, grated coconut and sunflower seeds

LUNCH
baked sweet potato with cottage cheese and green salad with avocado and peppers

DINNER
roast vegetables, to include acorn squash, bulb fennel and asparagus, topped with chickpeas and flavoured with cumin and chilli; mixed salad with dressing flavoured with tomato paste

Selenium, while obviously not a new mineral,
was relatively overlooked until 1957, when it was more fully
researched. Selenium is found in the soil and although plants do not
use selenium it is incorporated into their structure and so is available
to us via plant-based foods. It is also found in seafood, because the
marine vegetation on which fish partially feed is rich in selenium.
Research suggests that it is lacking in a modern Western diet, mainly
due to soil depletion. Human beings use selenium throughout the
body, but the highest levels are found in the liver, kidneys, spleen,
pancreas and testes.

As a trace element, selenium is essential in very small amounts,
while toxicity can occur at relatively low levels of around 1,000µg daily.
Taking supplementation should therefore be closely monitored as this
figure is relatively easy to exceed. While the recommended target
intake is 75µg for men and 60µg for women, therapeutic intake levels of
200µg appear to be necessary to produce beneficial results.

✔ Friends	✗ Foes
• There is a lack of scientific data on the inter-relation between selenium and other nutrients in the body. However, it would appear that **Vitamin E** has a beneficial effect on selenium levels.	• **Iron and copper deficiencies** interfere with metabolic pathways that involve selenium.

SEE ALSO

Vitamin C *p24*   Vitamin E *p28*   Copper *p54*   Iron *p58*   Fighting the Ageing Process *p100*
Boosting the Immune System *p106*   Maintaining Heart Health *p128*   Maintaining General Skin Health *p136*

How does the body use it?

Selenium is now widely recognized as an important antioxidant, primarily for its role in reducing potentially damaging oxidizing free radicals to harmless substances such as water. To date, no less than five selenium-dependent glutathione antioxidants have been identified. It also plays a particularly important role in protecting developing sperm from oxidative damage. As well as its own antioxidant activity, research has shown that selenium plays a part in recycling other antioxidants, such as vitamin E, vitamin C and glutathione. Unsurprisingly, it is becoming increasingly accepted that selenium is an important cancer-protective nutrient.

Insufficient selenium can reduce thyroid function because the reaction converting the thyroid hormone T4 into its active form of T3 is selenium-dependent.

Selenium is essential for an efficient immune system, displaying anti-bacterial and anti-viral properties and, combined with vitamin E, it promotes anti-inflammatory pathways. Selenium can therefore play a role in promoting skin health, particularly where acne, eczema and psoriasis, and herpes are concerned. It may also be helpful in chronic inflammatory conditions, such as lupus and arthritis.

There is still plenty of research needed on selenium to identify further its different enzymatic activities throughout the body.

WHAT ARE THE SIGNS OF GETTING TOO LITTLE?

Early deficiency signs include fatigue and muscle weakness, while white nail beds could also be an indicator. Long-term deficiency could lead to heart disease, cancer, immune problems and various chronic inflammatory conditions. It is possible that deficiency during pregnancy could lead to birth defects.

IS IT POSSIBLE TO GET TOO MUCH?

It is – if you eat foods that are rich sources of selenium, then any supplementation should be undertaken under the supervision of an appropriate nutrition expert. Ideally intake should not exceed 200µg from all sources.

What are the best food sources?

Because the selenium content of food is entirely dependent on its uptake from the soil, good food sources depend as much on where the foods were grown as on the nature of the food itself.

If the animals have been fed a diet sufficiently high in selenium, offal is a good source, particularly kidneys and liver. Herring, halibut, cod, salmon, sole, mackerel, lobster, scallops and prawns are also potentially good sources.

Brazil nuts, walnuts, cashew nuts, sesame seeds, oats, barley, brown rice, chicken, skimmed milk, kidney beans, onions and button mushrooms can be good sources.

A day's Supereating

BREAKFAST
scrambled egg with prawns on wholemeal toast, scattered with crushed Brazil nuts

LUNCH
smoked herring pâté with wholemeal bread, radishes and celery on the side

DINNER
grilled chicken breast served with brown rice and sautéed button mushrooms

Sodium is a mineral commonly found as the brittle crystals of sodium chloride, known as salt. Salt is found in abundance in the seas and oceans as well as in underground deposits that were formed by the evaporation of sea water. It has been recognized for thousands of years, with early trading routes established for salt transportation. Salt was so important to early civilizations that not only were taxes levied on it but it was considered as precious as gold.

Sodium is found in all living organisms and is an essential mineral. In the human body, 55% of our stores of it are found together with chloride in blood plasma and the fluid surrounding cells. About 40% of our sodium is found in bones and the rest within our organs.

Sodium is one of the very few nutrients that we consistently consume in quantities above the minimum daily requirement. As salt enhances the flavour of food, it is often used too liberally.

What are the best food sources?

Sodium is found in all living organisms and the best way to obtain it is from fresh foods, raw or lightly cooked and seasoned using herbs and spices, rather than adding extra salt. Fish is an obviously good source but red meat and poultry all contain sodium. Vegetables, particularly sea vegetables, all provide sodium, as do fruit, avocados and squashes. Dairy foods and cheese are high in sodium. Eggs contain sodium. Nuts and seeds in their natural form are quite low in sodium.

✔ Friends

• The message about sodium is that we consistently consume too much and it really needs no enhancement. The only times we may have increased requirements are during prolonged endurance exercise and working in very humid climates. In such extremes it is a simple process to consume salt and other electrolytes in a solution.

• Sodium needs to be in balance with other electrolytes, particularly **potassium**. It is interesting that most food in its natural form contains less sodium than potassium, often around half as much. Our modern Western diets have completely reversed this ratio.

✗ Foes

• It is possible to have low sodium in **very humid climates**, particularly when exercising heavily, because it will be lost in sweat.

• **Prolonged diarrhoea** may decrease levels.

• **Prolonged intense exercise**, such as running a marathon, may result in loss of sodium.

• The functions of sodium are mainly disrupted by **consuming too much salt**. This is found in all processed foods, packaged foods, canned foods, smoked meats, cooking processes and being added to food at the table. Serious culprits are snacks, such as crisps, salted nuts, etc.

Potassium *p66*   **Improving Digestive Health** *p118*   **Maintaining Heart Health** *p128*

How does the body use it?

The most important role of sodium is as an electrolyte. It works closely with other electrolytes, such as potassium and chloride, to regulate fluid levels in the body, which it does by activating a pump that lets water and nutrients into cells, while potassium pumps waste products out of cells. This fluid control is a vital part of our feedback mechanism for maintaining a healthy blood pressure.

Sodium electrolytes are also important for sending electrical messages throughout the nervous system, making it important for muscle contraction and nervous function. It also plays a role in nerve pain.

Sodium plays a role in digestion because it can help with the absorption of nutrients in the intestines and the chloride found in salt is used to make hydrochloric acid, which is vital for digestion in the stomach.

WHAT ARE THE SIGNS OF GETTING TOO LITTLE?
Sodium is found in all foods and our body is constantly adjusting concentrations, so chronically low sodium is rare. The signs of moderately low salt levels include fatigue, confusion and headaches, muscle cramps and nausea.

IS IT POSSIBLE TO GET TOO MUCH?
It is very easy to get too much sodium, partly because our metabolism is geared to retaining sodium while it easily excretes potassium, and partly because our Western diet is typically far too high in salt. We are recommended to eat no more than 6g of salt per day (2.5g sodium) but, on average, we are eating around 10g (about 4g of sodium). In reality, we could eat less than 6g, the minimum bodily requirement being 1.5g.

High levels of sodium lead to water retention and high blood pressure, and are associated with loss of elasticity in the walls of blood vessels, known as 'hardening of the arteries'.

As excess sodium can trigger the loss of calcium, bone thinning and osteoporosis can also be signs that we are getting too much. This close relationship with calcium means that excess salt can also contribute to the formation of kidney stones.

A day's Supereating

BREAKFAST
plain yoghurt, fresh fruit, mixed seeds, oat flakes

LUNCH
sweet potato and onion frittata flavoured with cumin and fresh coriander, mixed salad

DINNER
chicken stir-fried with ginger and other spices, pak choy and peppers, brown rice cooked in stock and flavoured with onion, cinnamon and cloves

Note: all the above will provide flavours that don't need additional salt while providing good levels of potassium

Sulphur

Sulphur is a bright yellow mineral that has been used medicinally for thousands of years – wounded Trojan soldiers were reputed to have used sulphur baths for healing their wounds and spa towns have long capitalized on their sulphur-rich spa waters to attract those looking to cure aches and pains of all kinds. Since the advent of antibiotics and other medications, sulphur has been largely overlooked therapeutically, yet it is found in every living cell and is the third most abundant mineral found in the human body, accounting for about 1% of our body weight. Despite its abundance, we need only trace amounts of this essential mineral.

✔ Friends

• An important metabolic pathway that uses sulphur is heavily dependent on **folate, vitamins B6 and B12.**

✘ Foes

• Because sulphur is predominantly found incorporated in amino acids (the building blocks of proteins) it is possible that **a diet that is vegan, or low in animal protein** may be low in sulphur.
• **High levels of zinc** can suppress sulphur levels.

What are the best food sources?

There are many foods that are good sources of sulphur, including all meat, poultry and fish. Eggs are an excellent source. Vegetable sources include onions, garlic, cabbage, Brussels sprouts, beans and peas.

SEE ALSO

Vitamin B6 *p40*   Folic Acid *p44*   Vitamin B12 *p46*   Zinc *p74*   Eating for Greater Energy *p124*
Maintaining Heart Health *p128*   Maintaining General Skin Health *p136*

How does the body use it?

A large proportion of sulphur in our bodies is incorporated in connective tissue; so skin, muscles, tendons and ligaments, hair and nails all benefit from the sulphur in our diet. For example, the protein keratin, which is found in hair, nails and the epidermis of our skin, contains 4% sulphur.

Sulphur acts as a detoxifier, being incorporated by the body into an important detoxifying antioxidant. It also plays an important role in protecting our cardiovascular systems, where it has a cholesterol-lowering effect on the blood. Sulphur compounds can also have an anti-parasite action.

As those who have used sulphur spas have found, sulphur helps reduce the pain and swelling in joints. This is because it appears to inhibit enzymes that encourage cartilage destruction and increase levels of synovial fluid (the gel-like membrane that lines our joints).

We also need sulphur for the formation of energy from glucose, fats and proteins.

WHAT ARE THE SIGNS OF GETTING TOO LITTLE?
Deficiencies are extremely rare due to the abundance of sulphur in most diets.

Because of its importance in connective tissue, the initial signs of sulphur deficiency will show in the skin, hair, nails and joints. So, dry skin, loss of skin elasticity, eczema, thinning hair, and brittle and slow-growing nails could all respond to better sulphur levels. Musculoskeletal disorders such as painful joints, back pain and arthritis can be signs of low sulphur.

High cholesterol and cardiovascular disease can also both be related to sulphur deficiency.

IS IT POSSIBLE TO GET TOO MUCH?
There are no records of toxicity from food sources.

A day's Supereating

BREAKFAST
scrambled or poached egg

LUNCH
mixed salad of broad beans and peas with a garlic dressing.

DINNER
grilled steak on stir-fried red cabbage with red onions

Zinc is not a newcomer, of course, but was only really researched from the 1960s onwards.

Despite the fact that zinc oxide has been used in baby barrier and other healing creams for many years, it is only since then that we have begun to understand how vital zinc is to hundreds of processes in the body. This is because zinc, a trace mineral needed in milligram quantities, was only measurable using highly accurate scientific instruments that became available in the late 60s.

Although widely used throughout the body, zinc is not actually stored, therefore it is highly dependent on dietary intake. Approximately 2g of zinc is contained in the body, but the pool of available zinc is small, with a rapid turnover. Concentrations of zinc are highest in muscles and bones, with significant levels being found in the skin, eyes, liver, kidneys, pancreas, adrenal glands and the prostate in men.

What are the best food sources?

Adequate amounts of zinc in the soil are necessary for plant uptake, so good food sources often depend on where it was raised or grown rather than on the food variety.

The most available form of zinc comes from protein, so meat, poultry, game, liver, eggs and seafood (particularly oysters) are all good sources. For vegetarians, cheese, yoghurt, beans, nuts, seeds, oats, brown rice, wheatgerm, pumpkin, seaweed and peas are good sources but the zinc is less absorbable.

In today's Western diets, high in processed foods, zinc levels may be very low. This is because food processing and refining (such as milling and canning) reduces zinc levels. Add to this the problem of zinc-depleted soils, a high-sugar diet, excess alcohol intake and high levels of phytic acid in vegetarian sources of zinc and you very quickly have a recipe for a zinc-depleted diet.

✔ Friends

• **Vitamin B6** increases zinc absorption.
• **Cysteine** is important for the synthesis of zinc transport molecules.
• **Histidine** can improve absorption by altering the pathways.

✗ Foes

The following can impair the absorption of zinc from food:
• **Phytates**, found in bran, legumes, some nuts and seeds.
• **Cellulose**, found in leafy plants.
• **High levels of folic acid.**
• **High levels of calcium, phosphorus, copper and iron intake**, because they all compete for the same binding sites to carry them across the gut wall.
• **Alcohol** increases the urinary excretion of zinc.
• **Sugar** increases the requirement for zinc.
• **Smoking** increases the need for antioxidants and will deplete zinc stores.

SEE ALSO

Vitamin C *p21*   Vitamin B6 *p40*   Boosting the Immune System *p106*   Maintaining General Skin Health *p136*

How does the body use it?

Zinc may be a trace mineral, but in terms of its importance it punches well above its weight and is critical for many aspects of health.

Its primary use is enzymatic, with approximately 100 different enzymes being zinc-dependent. In this role it is active in virtually every area of the body.

Zinc is well recognized for its role in supporting immune function and zinc levels are very important for a healthy thymus, often called the master gland of the immune system. Zinc increases resistance to infection and is commonly taken in conjunction with vitamin C when dealing with coughs, colds and flu.

Zinc is also a major antioxidant nutrient, protecting from free radical damage, as well as playing a role in DNA coding and protein synthesis, thereby optimizing healthy cell regeneration and healing. As a transporter of vitamin A, it maintains healthy skin and eyes.

Zinc is also known for its role in maintaining healthy sex organ function and high concentrations are found both in semen and the prostate gland.

Less widely known are its roles in insulin storage and activity, its importance for cognitive function and the importance of zinc levels for a healthy heart and thyroid function.

This seems an impressive repertoire for a mineral with a recommended daily intake of a mere 9.5mg for men and 7mg for women.

WHAT ARE THE SIGNS OF GETTING TOO LITTLE?
Deficiency signs for a mineral with such a wide range of uses are obviously quite varied. An early sign of zinc deficiency is an impaired sense of taste and smell, while white flecks in the nail may be another sign. Slow wound healing, frequent cold and flu infections and skin problems are other warning signals. Low zinc levels can also result in male infertility due to low sperm count and delayed infant cognitive development as well as impaired blood glucose handling. Zinc levels have also been shown to be low in some cases of rheumatoid arthritis.

IS IT POSSIBLE TO GET TOO MUCH?
It is highly unlikely that toxic levels of zinc could be reached through food alone.

A day's Supereating

BREAKFAST
glass of cider vinegar in hot water with a very little honey, live yoghurt mixed with fromage frais, mixed seeds, soaked apricots

LUNCH
seafood salad mixed with green peas and scattered with parsley; or a dozen oysters with a side salad

DINNER
grilled peppered venison steak with turnip and mustard mash and cauliflower sautéed with tomato paste, garlic and olive oil

Bioflavonoids

Bioflavonoids (often just called flavonoids) are a very diverse array of beneficial compounds found in fruits and vegetables. Initially known as 'vitamin P', they were first discovered in 1938 by the Nobel Prize-winning Hungarian scientist, Dr. Albert Szent-Györgyi and we still have much to learn about them. Under the umbrella term 'flavonoids' sits a wide range of plant chemicals (or phytochemicals) including flavonols, flavones, isoflavones, anthocyanins, anthocyanidins and saponins, many of which can be divided again into the over 4,000 single flavonoids so far identified. Members of one or other of the flavonoid families are found in all plant forms. Most of them are colourless, but some are highly coloured and are the compounds that give fruit and vegetables their bright colours.

What are the best food sources?

Virtually all plants (vegetables, fruits, herbs and spices, beans and grains) contain bioflavonoids.

Berries and red grapes are an excellent source of anthocyanins and proanthocyanidins.

Green tea contains catechins.

Both black and white tea are very potent sources of flavanols.

Buckwheat contains rutin.

Soya, kidney beans, peas and lentils contain isoflavones.

Red and yellow onions and shallots contain quercetin.

The white pulp of oranges contains hesperetin.

Parsley, thyme, oregano and celery contain flavones.

Citrus fruit juices are high in flavanones.

Onions, kale, leeks and broccoli contain flavonols.

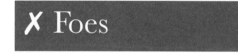

✔ Friends

Although we still have a vast amount to learn about all phytochemicals, including bioflavonoids, it seems logical to assume that they will work better together than in isolation.

✗ Foes

- **Processing and cooking** have a very negative impact on bioflavonoid levels.

How does the body use them?

The sheer numbers of different chemical compounds involved explains why we still know relatively little about flavonoids' role in human health. It seems clear, however, that in common with most phytochemicals, flavonoids act primarily as antioxidants, giving our cells protection from oxidative damage. They can also have an effect on cell signalling, which means that they will play a role in regulating cell growth and death. These two actions suggest that flavonoids could be significant in the prevention of cancer.

Another important role for flavonoids is the regulation of our inflammatory pathways. While inflammation is the body's natural response to damage, it needs to be strictly controlled to prevent an over-reaction from the immune system.

There appears to be a very close relationship between vitamin C function and flavonoids. Again, this was first discovered by Dr. Szent-Györgyi, who found that vitamin C worked more effectively when combined with flavonoids. This relationship gives flavonoids an important role in cardiovascular health.

Some flavonoids have antibacterial properties, giving them a direct role in the treatment of bacterial infections such as herpes and e. coli.

WHAT ARE THE SIGNS OF GETTING TOO LITTLE?
The current UK government recommendation to eat five portions of fruit and vegetables a day is closely linked to the levels of phytochemicals that this will provide. Too little has been shown to lead to many chronic diseases, including heart disease, high cholesterol, diabetes and some cancers.

IS IT POSSIBLE TO GET TOO MUCH?
Some flavonoids can cause a few problems. While teas are a good source of flavanols, black tea isn't the best source due to the caffeine content, and so relying on black tea for flavanols can lead to caffeine-related issues. Grapefruit juice contains a flavonoid called naringin that can disrupt liver detoxification pathways and disrupt certain medications.

A day's Supereating

BREAKFAST
buckwheat porridge with yoghurt and mixed berries, and a cup of green tea

LUNCH
salad of grated beetroot, red cabbage, sliced red onion and orange segments topped with feta cheese and mixed seeds

DINNER
red rice and yellow split pea casserole with onions and garlic and celery, steamed broccoli and a glass of red wine or red grape juice.

Note: these suggestions will provide a wide range of different bioflavonoids

Carotenoids is the name
given to a group of fat-soluble nutrients which are
generally the pigments that give both fruit and
vegetables their yellow, orange and red colours,
but also occur in birds and fish (flamingos and
salmon are obvious examples given their natural
colour). There are more than 600 carotenoid
compounds, some of which are very familiar, like
beta-carotene (which many people are aware of as
it is found in carrots and peppers, see vitamin A,
page 22) while others are lesser known and are the
subject of ongoing research. They are defined by
their chemical structure and the most commonly
occurring in our diets are alpha-, beta- and
gamma-carotene, beta-cryptoxanthin, lutein,
lycopene and zeaxanthin.

What are the best food sources?

Foods that are coloured yellow, orange or red provide the best
sources of most of the carotenoids, while green leafy vegetables
also provide some.

Carrots and sweet potato, spinach and kale, peaches and
apricots provide beta-carotene.

Carrots, pumpkins and red and yellow peppers provide alpha-
carotene.

Pumpkin, red peppers and orange-coloured fruit provide
cryptoxanthin.

Tomatoes, particularly processed, as in paste or tinned, are the
best source of lycopene.

Leafy greens such as kale and spinach as well as peas and
corn provide lutein and zeaxanthin.

Salmon, prawns and other seafoods are a good source of
astaxanthin.

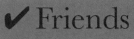

✔ Friends

• Because they are fat-soluble,
carotenoids are **better absorbed when
eaten with dietary fat.** It appears that
as little as 2–3g of fat in a meal will
facilitate absorption.
• Interestingly, **processing can
enhance the absorption** of some
carotenoids, particularly lycopene from
tomatoes.

✘ Foes

• **Unabsorbable fat** disrupts carotenoid
absorption, therefore functional foods
that lower cholesterol by including
unabsorbable fat will measurably
decrease blood levels of these vital
antioxidants.

How does the body use them?

The most widely understood role of carotenoids is as a precursor to vitamin A, which simply means that they are converted into a usable form of vitamin A in the body.

Since carotenoids are fat-soluble, they circulate in the blood with cholesterol and other fats. This has led to scientific research on their relationship with both heart disease and hardening of the arteries, and it appears that carotenoids can provide some protection against these conditions.

The carotenoids lutein and zeaxanthin are found in high concentrations in the retina of the eye, where they provide protection against damage from light. Research is ongoing into their probable role providing protection against cataract formation.

Studies are showing that carotenoids reduce the risk of various cancers: such as lung cancer (a broad spectrum of carotenoids) and prostate cancer (lycopene). Carotenoids play an important role in signalling from cell to cell and it is this that may give them an associated role in preventing cellular mutations. It seems likely that they also are very important for the female reproductive system, where very high levels are found.

WHAT ARE THE SIGNS OF GETTING TOO LITTLE?
Again, the current UK government recommendation to eat five portions of fruit and vegetables a day reflects the many nutrients, including phytochemicals, that this would naturally provide. A diet low in these antioxidant nutrients has been shown to lead to many chronic diseases, including heart disease, high cholesterol, diabetes and some cancers.

IS IT POSSIBLE TO GET TOO MUCH?
Some carotenoids in high levels may cause a yellow discoloration of the skin, but this will disappear when the intake is reduced. Both carotene and lycopene can cause this, and it may occur at lower levels with lycopene.

There have been studies that have shown that long-term high dose supplementation of beta-carotene by smokers may pose a risk of lung cancer.

A day's Supereating

BREAKFAST
cantaloupe melon, followed by yoghurt with mixed seeds and papaya

LUNCH
tomato and red pepper soup, rye bread drizzled with olive oil

DINNER
salmon on a purée of carrot and sweet potato, together with kale softened in olive oil with garlic

Note: these suggestions will provide a wide range of different carotenoids, cooked and with a little dietary fat to improve absorption

Glucosinolates is

the collective term for a group of plant chemicals present in the brassica family of vegetables, which includes cabbage, cauliflower and broccoli. These sulphur-containing compounds are often responsible for the bitter and hot taste of such vegetables, and found in condiments such as mustard and horseradish they help give our foods a more interesting flavour.

Glucosinolates can only be used by the body once they have been broken down by enzymes that are released either when foods containing glucosinolates are crushed or chewed or by the action of bacteria in our colon. Research into this class of phytochemical is new and ongoing, so we still have much to learn. Currently there are two derivatives of glucosinolates that have been highlighted for their therapeutic properties and these are isothiocyanates and indole-3-carbinol.

✔ Friends

• **Gut bacteria** can produce the enzyme to break down glucosinolates, so healthy gut bacteria are important for effective use of this compound. **Probiotics** and **miso** are therefore useful.

✗ Foes

• **Cooking, particularly in water,** can leach glucosinolates from foods, as well as destroying the enzyme that breaks down glucosinolates to their active forms.

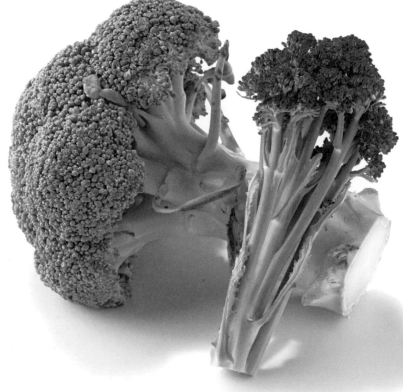

How does the body use them?

The most important role for isothiocyanates is in supporting liver detoxification pathways. They also help to regulate cell division and repair, as well as blocking the growth of damaged or mutant cells.

Indole-3-carbinol is also closely involved in aiding liver detoxification pathways, particularly those relating to oestrogen. Again, it plays an important role in blocking growth of damaged or mutant cells.

It is becoming clear that these compounds may also help prevent different cancers, including colon, stomach, lung and breast cancers, but research is still being undertaken to confirm these properties.

WHAT ARE THE SIGNS OF GETTING TOO LITTLE?
As with other phytochemical families, the current government recommendation to eat five portions of fruit and vegetables a day reflects the levels of phytochemicals that this will provide. A diet low in these antioxidant nutrients has been shown to lead to many chronic diseases including heart disease, high cholesterol, diabetes and some cancers.

IS IT POSSIBLE TO GET TOO MUCH?
There is evidence that eating large quantities of raw brassica vegetables can suppress thyroid function – these are included in a group of foods known as 'goitrogens' (see Iodine, page 56).

What are the best food sources?

Brassicas are the best source of glucosinolates.

Brussels sprouts, turnip, Savoy cabbage, kale, watercress and broccoli together will provide the full spectrum of glucosinolates.

Eating seed sprouts of the above (such as the old favourites 'mustard and cress') would give extra-high levels of glucosinolates.

A day's Supereating

BREAKFAST
live yoghurt, toasted oats and fresh fruit (to improve gut bacteria balance and thereby ensure good breakdown of glucosinolates)

LUNCH
sweet potato with cottage cheese (a fermented food that supports gut bacteria balance), a salad of shredded red and white cabbage and watercress in a horseradish and yoghurt dressing

DINNER
sautéed turkey or chicken breasts in mustard sauce, with steamed turnip cubes and steamed Brussels sprouts

Note: these suggestions will provide the full range of glucosinolates with the best possibility of including the necessary enzymes

Organosulphides is a collective

name for another group of plant chemicals, those that are naturally occurring in the onion family. Organosulphides are probably more readily recognized by another of their names, allium compounds; it is these important chemicals that give all members of the onion family their pungency.

Plants are our primary source of these important sulphur compounds, because they can synthesize inorganic sulphur into organic forms that we can use. Garlic is the most widely studied family member and its health benefits have been recognized across all cultures for many centuries. However, other members of the family should not be ignored, from the humble chive to leeks and red, yellow and white onions.

What are the best food sources?

Garlic, onions, leeks are all high in organosulphides, but garlic has had the most research carried out on it. Chives contain low levels of organosulphides.

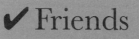

✔ Friends

• **Crushing garlic** induces the release of enzymes to activate the sulphur compounds. It is recommended that garlic be crushed and left to stand for 10 minutes prior to cooking to preserve active organosulphide compounds.

✗ Foes

• **Cooking, particularly by microwave,** can neutralize the beneficial effects of organosulphides.

How does the body use them?

Garlic may not ward off blood-seeking vampires, but it certainly protects the blood. Organosulphides have been shown to lower cholesterol levels by inhibiting its formation in the liver, they can also reduce plaque formation in blood vessels. Organosulphides have been shown to reduce the 'clumping' of red blood cells, thereby keeping blood flowing more freely. They also have an anti-inflammatory action that inhibits inflammatory white blood cell production.

Organosulphides can protect against the development of cancer, particularly in the stomach and colon. It seems that there are several mechanisms at work here: they help with two different detoxification pathways in the liver, so preventing the formation of cancer cells; they inhibit the proliferation of damaged cells, allowing time for repair, and they encourage the destruction of cells that are beyond repair. Through their action in the liver, organosulphides also play a significant role in antioxidant protection.

Garlic organosulphides are reputed to have anti-microbial properties that are particularly active in the colon.

It is not clearly understood how organosulphides are absorbed, but crushing or chewing garlic very quickly releases enzymes that react to produce sulphur compounds that appear to be metabolized extremely easily by the body, the only measurable traces of which are on the breath!

WHAT ARE THE SIGNS OF GETTING TOO LITTLE?
Again, the current Government recommendation to eat five portions of fruit and vegetables a day reflects the levels of phytochemicals this provides. A diet low in these antioxidant nutrients has been shown to lead to many chronic diseases, including heart disease, high cholesterol and some cancers.

IS IT POSSIBLE TO GET TOO MUCH?
Organosulphides from garlic produce body and breath odour, although these are both harmless. Some people may be sensitive to all plants in the allium family and can experience heartburn, abdominal pain, nausea, vomiting, flatulence and diarrhoea. High levels of supplementation may induce uncontrolled bleeding, particularly in conjunction with blood-thinning medication.

A day's Supereating

BREAKFAST
live yoghurt, toasted oats, seeds and fresh fruit (this will not provide organosulphides because for most of us the thought of garlic or onions at breakfast is a bit too much, but it will help support a healthy digestive tract for the absorption of all phytonutrients through the day)

LUNCH
roast mixed vegetables: onions, peppers, tomatoes, courgettes, drizzled after cooking with oil, crushed garlic and chopped chives

DINNER
grilled lean lamb steaks that have been marinated in olive oil, crushed garlic and white wine vinegar; leeks à la grecque (braised with brown rice, olive oil, garlic and tomato purée)

Note: these suggestions will provide a broad range of organosulphides, prepared to ensure absorption and utilization

Phyto-oestrogens are plant

chemicals that can be converted by intestinal bacteria into compounds that mimic some of the effects of oestrogen. Studies of the specific benefits of phyto-oestrogens give inconclusive results, but they are considered to have some benefit in preventing hormone-related cancers (perhaps because they play a role in signalling systems between cells), protecting against cardiovascular disease and may play a role in improving bone density. Phyto-oestrogens have also been used to improve some of the symptoms of menopause.

There are different families of phyto-oestrogens:

LIGNANS are a widespread group of phyto-oestrogens found mainly in seeds (particularly flaxseeds and sesame seeds), whole grains and legumes.

ISOFLAVONES are compounds found in soya products, such as tofu, miso, tempeh, roasted soya beans, lentils, peas (isoflavones also come into the bioflavonoid group of phytonutrients, see page 76).

PHYTOSTEROLS is a collective term for the plant-derived compounds sterols and stanols that are very similar to cholesterol. Phytosterols can lower cholesterol levels and be protective against cardiovascular disease. Some studies suggest that phytosterols may also be protective against some cancers, such as prostate and breast cancers. Phystosterols are found in all plants, but the highest concentrations are found in extra-virgin seed and nut oils, particularly corn oil. Wheat germ is also an excellent source.

RESVERATROL is an antioxidant nutrient produced by various plants, but most notably the grapevine. Its most important health benefits include protection against the risk of blood clots, stroke and cardiovascular disease as well as being cancer preventative. It also appears to have a weak phyto-oestrogenic action, as well as regulating cell production. Resveratrol is found in grape skins, wine and grape juice, and also in blueberries, bilberries and cranberries. It is quite concentrated in full-bodied red wines.

SAPONINS are plant chemicals that get their name from soapwort, a plant with foaming properties that was historically used as soap. Saponins have been shown to control cholesterol by both preventing its absorption in the small intestine and by increasing excretion of waste cholesterol. Although saponins are found in many plants, it is alfalfa that provides the most beneficial saponins for humans. Chickpeas and soya beans also provide some saponins.

Some other phytonutrients in brief

BROMELAIN is an enzyme that helps break down protein. It can be useful for improving digestion, but also can be used to help break down debris around injured and arthritic joints. It has anti-inflammatory properties and has been used to treat swelling and sprains. It can decrease the risk of thrombosis and also reduces mucous, so helps ease congestion in bronchitis. Bromelain is found in pineapples.

CAPSAICIN is an alkaloid chemical that is the active component of various species of pepper. Recent research reveals that capsaicin can kill cancer cells. It is also used to increase circulation and when employed topically can provide pain relief. Capsaicin is found in peppers, chillies, chilli powder and in paprika.

COUMARINS are members of the lactone group of plant chemicals. They are important for their anticoagulant action and some, such as Warfarin, are used medicinally. They occur in almost every plant, but good sources are beans, fennel, parsley and citrus fruit.

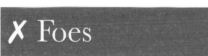

✔ Friends

- **Good intestinal flora**.
- **Probiotics**.
- A **high-carbohydrate** diet.

✘ Foes

- **Antibiotics**.

What are the best food sources?

For a good range of phyto-oestrogens, eat lots of whole grains, wheatgerm, legumes, soya products, alfalfa sprouts, seeds (especially sesame and flaxseeds), extra-virgin seed and nut oils, full-bodied red wine and grape juice, blueberries, bilberries and cranberries.

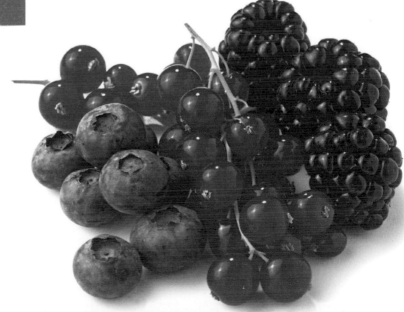

Probiotics is a term that has become much more familiar recently.

From the Greek word meaning 'for life', it is an umbrella term for beneficial bacteria present in fermented foods.

Our digestive systems contain a wide range of beneficial bacteria, the majority of which are found in the colon. In fact, our colon contains ten times more bacteria than there are cells in the rest of the body. These bacteria weigh in at 1kg and number more than 400 different species, with both beneficial and adverse effects on our health. A number of these species colonize the gut while others are transient, but they are all effectively competing for space, which is where probiotic foods can intervene, helping to promote the beneficial bacteria while suppressing those with adverse effects.

Man has used fermented foods for thousands of years and, while yoghurt and cheese are eaten worldwide, many ethnic fermented foods are also recognized for their health benefits: fermented cabbage in Germany and Eastern Europe; kefir (a fermented milk drink) in Russia; lassi (a fermented yoghurt drink) in India; fish in Korea, Sweden, Japan and Russia; and soya beans in Asia, to name but a few. At the beginning of the last century, a scientist called Elie Metchnikoff started to understand the scientific basis of these foods with the isolation of the bacterium *lactobacillus bulgaricus* – his paper called 'The Prolongation of Life' was published in this country in 1907. The use of antibiotics in the West resulted in a loss of interest in the benefits of such foods, but the new understanding of the down-side of antibiotic use has resulted in a resurgence of interest in the benefits of probiotic bacteria.

The most well-known of the probiotic bacteria are lactobacilli (*casei, acidophilus, plantarum, fermentum, reuteri* are lactobacillus species) found mainly in the small intestine, and bifidobacteria (*longum, lactis, infantis* are bifidobacterium species) found mainly in the colon, both of which are examples of colonizing bacteria. *Lactobacillus bulgaricus* is an example of a transient probiotic bacteria that does not adhere to the gut wall. Obviously, with over 400 species in the gut, the full list is long and complicated.

SEE ALSO

Vitamin K *p30*   Vitamin B family *p32–47*   Calcium *p50*   Boosting the Immune System *p106*
Improving Digestive Health *p118*   Maintaining General Skin Health *p136*

✔ Friends

• **Prebiotics**, that provide a food source for beneficial bacteria in the gut, will improve gut bacteria balance: these include oligosaccharides (found in bananas, tomatoes, onions and garlic), inulin (found in chicory and artichokes), resistant starch (found in pulses and whole grains).

• A level of at least 10 million bacteria in each helping is important in probiotic foods, due to the action of stomach acid.

✘ Foes

• Poor food choices (**too much sugar and yeast, too little fibre**) can have a detrimental effect on probiotic bacteria in the gut.

• **Age** can drastically reduce beneficial bacteria levels in the gut.

• **Stomach acid** will kill off many probiotic bacteria in fermented foods.

• **Some yoghurts** do not contain beneficial probiotic bacteria, they only contain the bacteria strains used for making the yoghurt.

• **Alcohol.**

• **Stress.**

• **Antibiotic use.**

How does the body use them?

Beneficial bacteria in the gut have an amazingly broad range of influence on health and, while we are beginning to understand many of these pathways, it seems that there is still much to be learned. A healthy balance of probiotic bacteria can crowd out pathogenic organisms; they ferment fibre that we cannot digest directly, forming short-chain fatty acids that keep the gut acidic and help maintain a healthy level of sugar and fats in the blood; they influence the uptake of calcium; they promote the movement of food through the gastrointestinal (GI) tract; they play a role in the formation of vitamin K and B vitamins; they metabolize bile acids, so play a role in liver support; they are protective against certain cancers, including colon cancer; they even show antioxidant properties.

From birth, *bifidobacteria infantis* is the first probiotic bacteria to colonize the infant gut and is obtained through mother's milk. These initial bacteria lay the foundation of a healthy immune system, and beneficial gut bacteria play a vital role in promoting a healthy immune response from birth throughout life. Although we do not fully understand precisely how gut bacteria interact with the immune system, it seems clear that they affect immune responses along the entire length of GI tract as well as preventing antigens (or molecules that provoke an immune response) from crossing the gut wall.

Probiotic bacteria have been used in the treatment of many diseases, including Crohn's disease, colitis, viral infections of the GI tract and infant diarrhoea. They are increasingly being used to prevent infection from so-called superbugs such as *clostridium dificile*; the transitory probiotic *saccharomyces boulardii* appears to be most effective here.

There is also increasing evidence that probiotic bacteria play a role in the treatment of conditions that are not apparently connected to the gut, such as attention deficit disorders and autism-related conditions, together with psoriasis and eczema.

It is not surprising, therefore, that beneficial gut bacteria can have an impact on virtually every aspect of health.

WHAT ARE THE SIGNS OF AN IMBALANCE?
The main symptoms of an imbalance of beneficial gut bacteria are bloating after meals and pain in the lower gut. Constipation and/or diarrhoea are also symptoms.

IS IT POSSIBLE TO GET TOO MUCH?
It may be possible to change the balance of gut bacteria too suddenly by taking high levels of a probiotic supplement, which could induce stomach pain and diarrhoea, but these symptoms are quickly reversed by reducing the dose.

What are the best food sources?

The best food sources of probiotic bacteria are fermented foods: kefir, sauerkraut, yoghurt, miso soup, tempeh and honey.

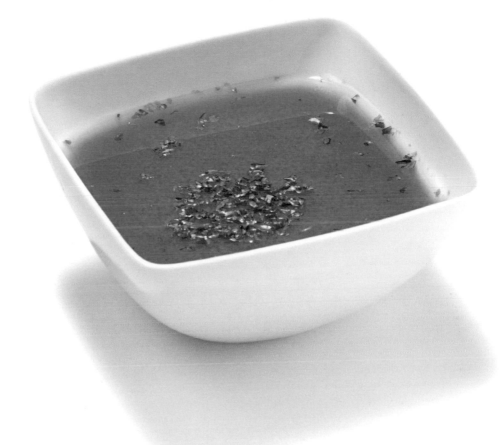

A day's Supereating

BREAKFAST

live yoghurt with toasted oats and sliced banana (providing both probiotics and prebiotics)

LUNCH

artichoke soup with a swirl of yoghurt and wholegrain bread (providing both probiotics and prebiotics)

DINNER

vegetable bean stew with garlic, onions and tomatoes (provides prebiotic foods)

Essential Fatty Acids are

the fats our body cannot make but needs for a wide variety of essential functions. There are two varieties of essential fatty acids (EFAs for short), omega-3 and omega-6. Another fatty acid, given the name of omega-9, can be made by the body, so is not strictly essential, however research is beginning to reveal how important omega 9 is for our health, hence its inclusion in the group. EFAs form part of every cell in the body and need to be eaten regularly.

The names given to fats can be very complicated and the terms 'saturated', 'unsaturated', 'polyunsaturated', 'omega-3', 'omega-6', 'hydrogenated' and 'trans fats' are bandied about by the food industry, dietitians and nutritionists alike, so it could be useful to try and explain some of these terms before going any further.

Whether fats are saturated, mono-unsaturated or polyunsaturated refers to the general chemical structure of the fat (which looks a little like a caterpillar) and whether all the links in the chains are firmly bound together (the tightly bound ones are known as 'saturated fats'), if there is one 'spare' link that is doubling up (mono-unsaturated fat) or if there are many of these spare links (polyunsaturated). How far down the chain these spare links occur, gives the fat its omega number (3, 6, 9, etc.).

Polyunsaturated fats, like most vegetable and nut oils, are liquid at any temperature; monounsaturated fats (like olive oil) are liquid at room temperature but solid when chilled; saturated fats (like butter and lard) are solid at room temperature.

It is the chemical structure of the fats, the bonds, which are easily affected by light and high heats. It is these damaged fats that are a health concern as they are a potential source of free radicals, short-lived substances that can alter chemical reactions within the body, which can lead to an increased risk of cardiovascular complications, some cancers and the visible signs of ageing. This is why we are advised to cook using olive oil or rapeseed oil (omega-3 and-6 fats) because they are more resilient to heat. Unexpectedly perhaps, butter is just as good as long as it's not allowed to burn, as butter is quite

SEE ALSO
Vitamin C *p24*   Vitamin E *p28*   Vitamin B3 *p36*   Vitamin B6 *p40*   Magnesium *p60*
Selenium *p68*   Zinc *p74*   Boosting the Immune System *p106*   Dealing with Stress *p112*
Maintaining Heart Health *p128*   Maintaining General Skin Health *p136*

stable at higher temperatures. Food processing can damage fats even further, particularly because processed foods are dependent on having a relatively long shelf-life. This has led to many commercial processes that make fats inert (or 'dead'), so they cannot react to light and heat. Hydrogenating, i.e. producing trans fats, deodorizing, superheating and bleaching are all processes that are used to give fats a longer shelf-life and make them more stable for use in the food industry. Sadly, these fats are not recognized by our bodies and therefore can disrupt hundreds of our metabolic pathways.

✔ Friends

- **Vitamin E** occurs naturally in foods containing EFAs because it works to protect these susceptible fats. Vitamin E has a similar effect on fats in our body, giving antioxidant protection.
- Other **antioxidants** keep EFAs healthy, including carotene, selenium and vitamin C.
- Effective absorption of EFAs depends on a **healthy gall bladder** to provide emulsifying agents.
- EFAs' pathways in the body depend on very specific essential nutrients: **vitamins B3, B6 and C, magnesium and zinc.**
- **Good storage:** seed oils need to be stored in dark glass bottles away from sunlight and heat; seeds need to be stored in the fridge; nuts should be kept in their shells until eaten and stored in a cool place.

✗ Foes

- As discussed above, the main disruption to EFAs is through **exposure to heat, light and food processing,** which damages them, turning them rancid.
- **Over-consumption of saturated fats** and commercially treated fats will affect the way we can use the essential fats.

How does the body use them?

There are two main functions of essential fatty acids.

Firstly, they link with proteins to make cell membranes, which means that essential fatty acids are found literally everywhere in our bodies. The cells of our nervous system, particularly the brain, are very concentrated in these fats.

Secondly, they form hormone-like substances called prostaglandins. These act a bit like thermostats, regulating many chemical reactions in our body, from immune responses to bone formation.

The first role of EFAs in cell formation is vital for the fluidity of cell membranes. If these are too rigid (too many saturated fats), then nutrients will have a problem crossing into cells, while at the same time toxins will not be eliminated effectively. The brain and nervous system are dependent on the right EFA balance, particularly for transmission of electrical messages along the nerves. They also play a role in the prevention of depression and are also vital for a healthy retina in the eye.

The most widely recognized role of prostaglandins is in the regulation of inflammation, giving EFAs an important role in the progression of inflammatory conditions such as rheumatoid arthritis, eczema and hay fever. Prostaglandins also play a role in relaxing the walls of blood vessels, so reducing blood pressure; they are important for the stimulation of uterine muscle contraction at childbirth; they play a role in bone formation; and they regulate the contraction of the muscles in the intestines.

EFAs have been widely researched in association with cardiovascular disease and it is recognized that they can reduce levels of fats circulating in the blood, particularly when this is linked to diabetes.

EFAs also play an important role in suppressing tumour formation, particularly in breast cancer. Their role in cell signalling may also be important here.

Dry skin, menopause and PMS symptoms, inflammatory bowel disease and attention deficit disorder can be ameliorated by a healthy intake of EFAs.

What are the best food sources?

The best food sources of beneficial EFAs are fish, nuts, seeds, avocados and their oils.

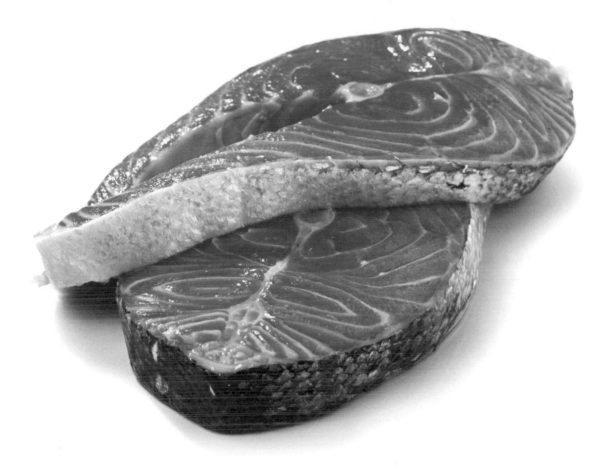

WHAT ARE THE SIGNS OF GETTING TOO LITTLE?
The first clinical signs of too little EFAs in the diet are a dry and scaly skin, brittle hair and nails, and constipation. Poor wound healing and frequent infections can also be related to low EFAs. Infants' and children's growth may be retarded. Problems with the nervous system may include depression, visual problems and nerve damage, while joint pains and poor physical endurance could also be related to low EFAs.

IS IT POSSIBLE TO GET TOO MUCH?
The most immediate sign of getting too many EFAs is loose stools, a symptom which is quickly reversible.

More serious problems may arise if someone is susceptible to easy bruising and bleeding, particularly if using blood thinning drugs such as Warfarin.

The anti-inflammatory actions of omega-3 fatty acids may suppress the immune system, which could be a problem for people with compromised immunity.

At-a-glance Summary of Nutrient Friends and Foes

	A	C	D	E	K	B1	B2	B3
Vitamin A				H				
Vitamin C								
Vitamin D								
Vitamin E		✔						
Vitamin K								
Vitamin B1							✔	✔
Vitamin B2						✔		✔
Vitamin B3						✔	✔	
Vitamin B5		✔				✔	✔	✔
Vitamin B6						✔	✔	✔
Biotin (B7)						✔	✔	✔
Folic Acid (B9)						✔	✔	✔
Vitamin B12						✔	✔	✔
Boron (B)								
Calcium (Ca)			✔/H					
Chromium (Cr)		✔						✔
Copper (Cu)		✗						
Iodine (I)	✔							
Iron (Fe)	✔	✔						
Magnesium (Mg)			✔					
Manganese (Mn)								
Phosphorus (P)			✔					
Potassium (K)								
Selenium (Se)				✔				
Sodium (Na)								
Sulphur (S)								
Zinc (Zn)								
Bioflavanoids								
Carotenoids								
Glucosinolates								
Organosulphides								
EFAs		✔		✔				✔
Probiotics								

This chart shows friends and foes only among the nutrient families; for the effects of other factors, such as food groups, special diets, bodily conditions etc., see the pages on the individual nutrients.

	B5	B6	Biotin	FA	B12	B	Ca	Cr	Cu
A									
C									
D						✔			
E									
K									
B1	✔	✔	✔	✔	✔				
B2	✔	✔	✔	✔	✔				
B3	✔	✔	✔	✔	✔				
B5		✔	✔	✔	✔				
B6	✔		✔	✔	✔				
(B7)	✔	✔		✔	✔				
(B9)	✔	✔	✔		✔				
B12	✔	✔	✔	✔					
(B)									
(Ca)									
(Cr)									
(Cu)							✗		
(I)									
(Fe)							✔/H		✔
(Mg)							✔/H/L		
(Mn)							H		H
(P)							✔/H		H
(K)									
(Se)									L
(Na)									
(S)		✔		✔	✔				
(Zn)		✔					H		H
Bioflav's									
Carot'ids									
Gluc'lates									
Organ'ides									
EFAs		✔							
Probiotics									

(continued overleaf)

At-a-glance Summary of Nutrient Friends and Foes (continued)

	I	Fe	Mg	Mn	P	K	Se	Na
Vitamin A		L						
Vitamin C								
Vitamin D								
Vitamin E							✔	
Vitamin K								
Vitamin B1			✔					
Vitamin B2								
Vitamin B3		✔						
Vitamin B5								
Vitamin B6								
Biotin (B7)								
Folic Acid (B9)								
Vitamin B12								
Boron (B)			✔					
Calcium (Ca)			✔/H			✔		
Chromium (Cr)								
Copper (Cu)		✔		✗	✗		✔	
Iodine (I)		✔/H					✔	
Iron (Fe)								
Magnesium (Mg)								
Manganese (Mn)		H	H		H	✔		
Phosphorus (P)		H	L					
Potassium (K)								
Selenium (Se)		L						
Sodium (Na)								H
Sulphur (S)								
Zinc (Zn)		H			H			
Bioflavanoids								
Carotenoids								
Glucosinolates								
Organosulphides								
EFAs			✔				✔	
Probiotics								

KEY - Friend: ✔ | Foe: ✗ | Foe when high: **H** | Foe when low: **L**

	S	Zn	Bio'oids	Car'oids	Glucos	Organos	EFAs	Probio's
Vitamin A		L						
Vitamin C								
Vitamin D								
Vitamin E								
Vitamin K								✔
Vitamin B1								✔
Vitamin B2								✔
Vitamin B3								
Vitamin B5								
Vitamin B6								
Biotin (B7)								✔
Folic Acid (B9)								
Vitamin B12								
Boron (B)								
Calcium (Ca)		✗					✔	✔
Chromium (Cr)								
Copper (Cu)		✗						
Iodine (I)								
Iron (Fe)		✗						✔
Magnesium (Mg)								
Manganese (Mn)		✗						
Phosphorus (P)								
Potassium (K)								
Selenium (Se)								
Sodium (Na)								
Sulphur (S)		H						
Zinc (Zn)								
Bioflavanoids			✔					
Carotenoids							✔	
Glucosinolates								✔
Organosulphides								
EFAs		✔		✔				
Probiotics								

Supereating
for Wellbeing

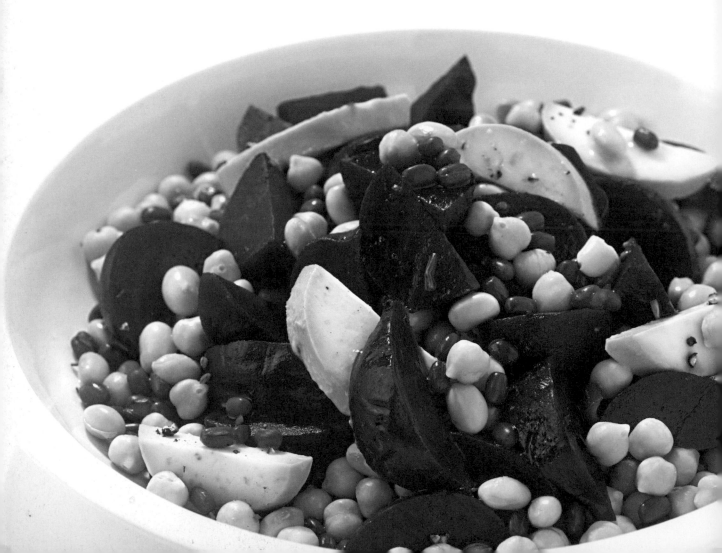

IT IS IN THIS CHAPTER THAT SUPEREATING COMES TO LIFE in a practical way, which is of course the only way that an eating plan can be successful. Hopefully, it is not too complicated and you will be able either to apply the advice in full, or to pick out the parts that work best for you. It may be that you already follow nutritional advice to help manage a condition or symptoms, but applying some of the principles of Supereating will offer a more robust and successful result.

Many issues have proven protocols that can alleviate symptoms or reduce the risk of illness. For example, the discomfort associated with arthritis can be ameliorated by reducing inflammation. From a nutritional standpoint, avoiding members of the nightshade family (such as potatoes, tomatoes, peppers, etc.) can help, as can getting plenty of the essential fats, mostly omega-3s. If we apply the Supereating approach, we can build on the proven benefits of these particular nutrients by improving the effectiveness of the nutrient in question. Using essential fats as an example, they have friends and foes as you can see in the last chapter. By ensuring that we get a lot of the friends, and by avoiding the foes, we can potentially improve on the old approach by simply enhancing the action of such essential fats and other nutrients.

As this book is an introduction to Supereating, introducing the principles involved, I have chosen a small number of health issues that are perhaps the most familiar ones. Certainly they are those that my clients ask about most often in consultations, and include advice on digestion, energy, combating stress, skin health, anti-ageing, heart health and immune boosting.

The guidelines I am proposing for these issues should offer a strengthened version of the established approach, and in the future these will be expanded. For now, however, I have identified the most important nutrients for each area and then shown how to maximize their benefits and minimize their foes. At the end of each section you will find an example of how to eat in the Supereating way for each area of health.

Fighting
the ageing process

GETTING OLDER DOES HAVE ITS BENEFITS, **but today's youth-orientated society does suggest that ageing is an affliction that we should avoid. The greatest compliment that one person can pay another is to say that they look great for their age, which implies that the recipient is looking after themselves well and it shows.**

Our cells replace themselves throughout our lives, but genetics play a role in how well we age, as every cell in the body will only replicate a finite number of times. The cells may replicate a few times or dozens of times, that number is genetically programmed, and once a cell stops replicating then what we think of as ageing manifests itself. Therefore, protecting the cells from damage, which means that they are then forced to replicate, or extending the life of a cell can, to some extent, slow down the ageing process. Aside from natural cell death (i.e. when a cell is programmed to self-destruct and replace itself with a new one), the cells can be damaged by a variety of factors, such as illness, injury and trauma.

It is widely believed that the actions of free radicals play a major role in damaging cells, and therefore counteracting them can hinder natural ageing. Free radicals are unpaired electrons that are looking for a home. When they find one, the biochemical make up of the new cell in which they have taken up residence is changed, making it unstable. This sounds very technical, but let me give you two examples that will make it far easier to picture.

Firstly, think of water, regular tap water. As you probably know, its chemical description is H_2O, which means that it comprises 2 atoms of hydrogen and 1 of oxygen. When apart, the 2 parts of hydrogen are stable, as they are in a pair,

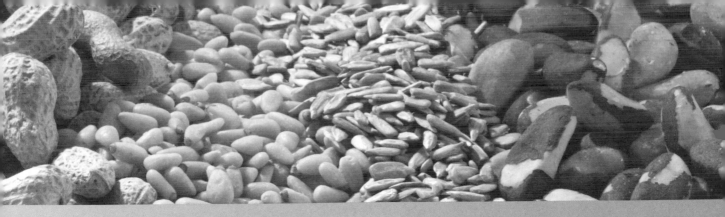

and the single atom of oxygen is looking for a home, and when it joins with the paired hydrogen atoms, water is formed. Now, we know that water is benign, so the result of the addition of the oxygen to the existing paired hydrogen atom is a good thing. However, not all pairings go quite so well, and the results can be damaging. For example, unpaired electrons (which are known as free radicals) can force themselves on to other already happily coupled electrons. This action changes the chemical structure into something that is potentially unstable, not like water at all.

In consultations, I often describe the damage caused by free radicals by asking my client to imagine a piece of fruit, perhaps a pear, cut in half and left in their kitchen for an hour. After a period of time the white flesh will turn brown, it has oxidized, much like rusting metal exposed to the elements for long periods. Had an antioxidant, like the vitamin C found in citrus juice, been poured on the fruit, then this would have slowed down the damage from the oxygen in the air. The juice would have acted as an antioxidant, and in much the same way nutrients that have antioxidant properties can protect cells from free radical damage.

Some sections of each cell are especially vulnerable to the actions of free radicals, notably the DNA (or deoxyribonucleic acid to give it its full name) and the outer layers of the cell. The DNA is vulnerable as its structure is like that of a ladder, the outer part of the ladder being linked by bonds. It's these bonds, or double bonds in fact, that are prone to free radical damage. These same double bonds exist in the outer layer of the cell, as it is mostly made of fats derived from the essential fats in the diet.

Free radicals are created by some day-to-day functions of the body, but also by other factors that are more related to lifestyle. The normal metabolism creates free radicals, like exhaust from a car engine, and so antioxidants are required daily, but this demand increases if we exercise, as we then create more free radicals. The immune system also creates free radicals as white blood cells do their work. (Other factors, such as smoking, exposure to ultraviolet light and the heavy metals we are increasingly exposed to in polluted environments are also sources of free radicals.)

The body produces substances of its own to combat free radicals, notably superoxide dismutase, known as SOD, and glutathione peroxidise (GP). Both are nutrient-dependent (SOD requires copper, zinc and manganese for its formation and GP relies on selenium). This is in addition to the nutrients our bodies use that have antioxidant effects of their own.

Antioxidant nutrients are to be found in many foods, but the majority are derived from fruits and vegetables. However, it's not all 'eat your greens', as antioxidants (resveratrol for example) are found in grape skins and seeds, which is the reason that red wine is able to be associated with good health. The same is true of chocolate, as the cocoa bean contains flavanols, which are noted for their antioxidant ability.

We have to be a little cautious here as there is an element of the old 'One-step' theory in this way of thinking. If grapes contain resveratrol, and red wine contains grapes, then should we assume that red wine is good for us? Well, to an extent that is true, but when we take into account that there is considerable

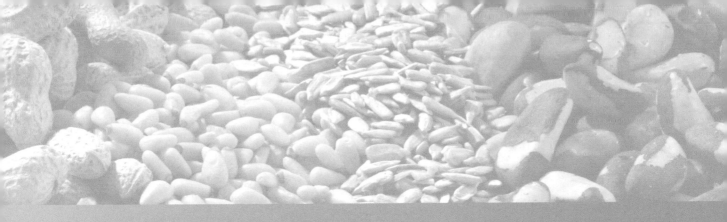

research into the detrimental effects of alcohol (even one glass a day), then should we get the antioxidants from wine or look elsewhere? Likewise, only the darkest chocolate can have a positive effect on our health, as all others are likely to contain refined sugars and fats, which to a large extent negate the benefits of the flavanols.

The theory of antioxidants is a well established one, but has been challenged from time to time. My own personal view is that the role of antioxidants may have been overstated and achieved a 'Holy Grail' status in some circles. Nonetheless, they are hugely important in combating free radicals and thus going some way to reducing the degradation of cells that goes hand in hand with getting older.

The free radical and antioxidant theory is also linked to cardiovascular disease (see pages 128–135) as free radicals can damage the lining of the veins and arteries. It is also associated with the formation of some forms of cancer, as the cells become damaged and replace themselves with mutant, or faulty, cells.

Nutrients for fighting ageing

Normal daily antioxidant requirements for combating free radical damage are taken into account with the general advice to consume at least five pieces of fruit and vegetables daily. However, with Supereating it is possible to maximize the action of these antioxidants.

nutrients and their role

Copper is involved with the body's production of free-radical-combating superoxide dismutase (SOD)

Zinc is involved with the body's production of SOD

Manganese is involved with the body's production of SOD

Selenium is involved with the body's production of free-radical-combating glutathione peroxidise (GP)

Vitamin A for its own antioxidant properties

Vitamin C for its own antioxidant properties

Vitamin E for its own antioxidant properties

Bioflavonoids for their own antioxidant properties

Carotenoids for their own antioxidant properties

A day's Supereating

BREAKFAST
fruit salad made with diced pineapple, apricots, kiwi fruit and grapefruit, topped with sesame seeds

MORNING SNACK
cashew nuts and raw mushrooms

LUNCH
salad of mixed beans (adzuki, soya, chickpeas), served with sliced avocado and beetroot

AFTERNOON SNACK
pecan nuts and chopped boiled egg

DINNER
grilled or tinned tuna served accompanied by roast leeks, butternut squash and steamed spinach, topped with pine nuts

✔ Friends	*foods to go for*	✘ Foes	*foods to avoid*
None	Liver, cashew nuts, sesame seeds, sunflower seeds, mushrooms, soya beans and adzuki beans (but see Foods to Avoid)	Excess zinc and vitamin C can reduce copper levels; excess fructose (fruit sugars)	• **Excess fructose,** limit fruit to 2 pieces a day but make up for this with plenty of vegetables
Vitamin B6 Protein	Seafood, chicken, oats, brown rice, pumpkin seeds	Excess cellulose & phytates High calcium intake Alcohol and refined sugar	• **Fruit juices** • **Low-fat** versions of regular foods; instead choose full-fat milk and butter used sparingly
Excessive supplementation of minerals, especially zinc, copper, magnesium, iron and calcium	Pineapple (but see Foods to Avoid), pecan nuts, pine nuts, soya nuts, sweet potato, spinach	Phytates and oxalates	• **Cholesterol-reducing foodstuffs** (plant sterols) • **Raw food** – eat vegetables steamed and not boiled
Iodine	Liver, halibut, cod, tuna, salmon, prawns, mushrooms, sole, mackerel, brown rice, onions, Brazil nuts, sesame seeds, cashew nuts	Low intake of copper and iron	• **Phytates** (such as cereal grains, legumes like chickpeas, beans and lentils, and plant tissue (Note: plant tissue includes all vegetables and so the importance of these for fibre and nutrient content has to be considered in relation to their benefit over the antagonistic properties of the phytates) should be minimized but not avoided as they are useful sources of fibre and other nutrients.
Protein Fat Zinc, iron	Eggs, liver, cheese, apricots, sweet potato, butternut squash, peppers (especially red and orange)	Plant sterols Low-fat diets	
Raw fruits and vegetables	Citrus fruits, kiwi fruit (but see Foods to Avoid), sweet potato, peppers	Excessive liquid intake as vitamin water-soluble Cooking	
Vitamin C Selenium	Avocados, almonds, peanuts, sunflower seeds, olive oil, eggs, tuna	Low-fat diets Plant sterols	
None	Citrus fruits (but see Foods to Avoid), green and white tea, red wine, dark chocolate, beetroot, onion, leeks	Dehydration	
Dietary fats	Carrots, spinach, kale, pumpkins, peppers, tomato, spinach, peas, peaches, apricots (but see Foods to Avoid)	Artificial fats	

Boosting
the immune system

WHEN WE THINK ABOUT THE IMMUNE SYSTEM, we do tend instantly to think just of coughs, colds and flu, but there are other far more serious situations, not least cancers, that are immune-related, and so supporting this system has enormous value.

The immune system is a complicated one, undoubtedly the most complex in the body. Challenges to the body are everywhere – on every surface, in the air and in our food and drink – and an efficient immune system has to work relentlessly to deal with threats on all fronts. When potential pathogens enter the body, the various elements of the immune system will deal with them, neutralizing and eliminating them. The immune system is always working, at times more forcefully than others, and there are several factors that can help enhance the efficiency of the immune response.

Given that the workings of the immune system could fill a huge tome in itself, it is appropriate here just to look at the basic elements of the system that are directly affected and supported by nutrients. The several types of immune cells

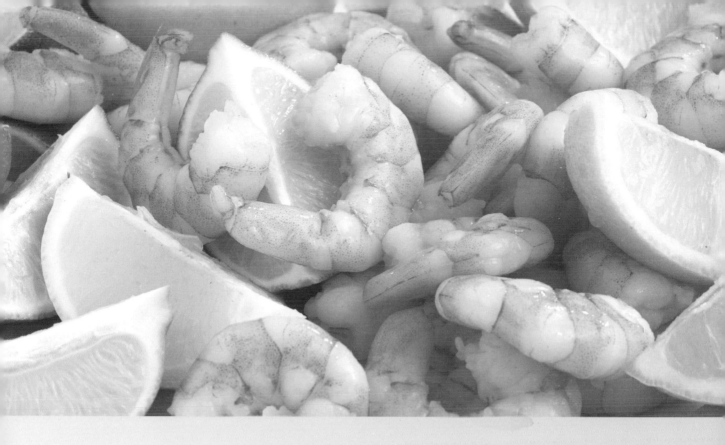

(listed overleaf) that are manufactured in a variety of places around the body all have different roles to play, but collectively they create an effective force that detects and deals with all manner of potentially damaging bacteria and viruses. Do remember that our own cells themselves can become damaged, and they need to be dealt with in much the same way as any other unwanted substance, so once a cell is damaged, the immune system works on neutralizing it and clearing it away.

In the past I have compared the variety of immune cells to a naval fleet, protecting an island (in this case, your body). It is an apt description, as some cells wander around looking for trouble – on patrol, if you like – while others have fixed positions that deal with passing pathogens.

The inflammatory response is an invaluable tool

by means of which the body identifies, isolates and mounts a concerted response to attack or damage. For example, imagine something quite mundane, albeit painful, like catching your finger in a door. Obviously we know that the finger will become red and swollen. This is often seen as a problem in itself, but it is in fact the repair and recovery process in action. Extra blood is directed to the damaged area, taking with it white blood cells that release various substances that counteract the damaged cells. The finger will be sore and painful and, as a result, you might be careful and avoid using it, which will further aid recovery.

Inflammation is a vital part of the immune response, but it is tightly controlled. The process is initiated by the correct triggers (damage or infection, for example) and then the process is halted when the stimulus is dealt with. It is when the immune system fails to switch off the inflammatory response that we can experience symptoms such as those associated with arthritis.

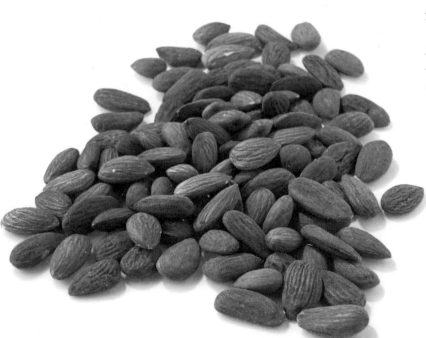

ISSUES THAT ADVERSELY AFFECT
THE IMMUNE SYSTEM
1 Being run down, sleep-deprived or stressed, which is why we tend to suffer from more infections when feeling generally low.
2 Diets of less than 1,200 calories per day.
3 High intake of saturated fats.
4 Excessive exercise.
5 Low intake of protein.

The main active components of the immune system

Complement

This is a protein found in the blood that is usually inactive, but when the immune system is challenged, it can improve – or complement – the action of immune cells.

Interferon

This is a fluid with mild anti-viral properties that is secreted by all tissue once it is under threat from a pathogen.

Red blood cells

These are produced in the bone marrow and are mainly used to carry oxygen and nutrients around the body while removing metabolic waste. Lozenge-like in shape, red blood cells have a smooth surface and concavities on either side to be able to attach themselves to compounds they want to transport through the bloodstream. Some are misshapen, however, and lack the ability to carry many nutrients so are less efficient. These misfit cells are increased through over-exercise, and also poor nutrition.

White blood cells (leukocytes)

There are many types of white blood cells, or leukocytes, and they have a very active job as the fighting men of the immune system. Each type of leukocyte has a slightly different role to play, but their production and action is closely linked to proper nutrition.

Neutrophils

Often the very first cells to be involved in defending against fungal and bacterial infections, these are involved in the process of inflammation, and have a phagocytic action, that is the ability to change shape and engulf the bacteria or virus, neutralizing it in the process. Neutrophils are fast-acting and short-lived, and their end product is pus.

Monocytes

Not unlike neutrophils but longer-lasting, these white blood cells are also phagocytic. They also act as carriers by taking particles of pathogens to T cells (see below) to trigger a reaction. Monocytes travel from the blood into the tissue, and are then known as macrophages.

Basophils

These cells release histamine, which is involved in the inflammatory response. Most of us are familiar with histamine, as it is well known in the allergic response.

Eosinophils

These white blood cells are also involved in the allergic reaction, and result in familiar issues such as hay fever and skin eruptions or hives. Eosinophils are also required to combat parasites, mostly found in the gastrointestinal tract.

Lymphocytes (B, T and NK cells)

The body's lymphatic system takes fluids from the blood stream to the tissues. In it, lymphocytes are produced. There are three main types of lymphocytes: B cells, which make the antibodies that will cling to pathogens; T cells, which detect and act against mutant cells or cells that have become cancerous or infected by a pathogen and, lastly, Natural Killer (NK) cells, which destroy other infected or cancerous cells.

Nutrients for immune boosting

There is a strong link between nutrients and the workings of specific immune cells. All nutrients are involved in the immune system, yet some seem to have a more direct role than others. Here we examine those that I believe to be the most important.

Using the Supereating approach, we can identify the key nutrients, their friends and foes, and thus the foods that will enhance their effect and those to avoid. We can thus formulate a Supereating plan that should provide the optimum ratio of nutrients.

A day's Supereating

BREAKFAST
plain yoghurt with pumpkin seeds and blueberries

MORNING SNACK
oatcake with cashew butter or salmon pâté

LUNCH
salad made with cooled steamed asparagus, mixed salad leaves, soft-boiled eggs, sliced yellow and red peppers, sprinkled with sesame seeds; dressing of plain yoghurt mixed with lemon juice, olive oil and crushed garlic

AFTERNOON SNACK
soft fruits mixed with flaked almonds

DINNER
grilled chicken or king prawns, served with steamed cauliflower, broccoli and brown rice

nutrients and their role

Vitamin A is involved with antibody production and cell replication (so that cells divide normally and do not mutate) and supports the thymus gland

Vitamin B6 works to support both B and T cells

Vitamin C has many roles to play in the immune system: it can increase antibody production and is a component of both interferon and complement

Vitamin E can increase the concentration of T cells

Zinc is required by the thymus gland in the manufacture of T cells

Selenium is involved in the action of both NK and T cells, also in the production of antibodies

Iodine stimulates NK cells

Bioflavonoids in the tissue trigger a response that works against carcinogens and thus have a potential role in warding off some cancers

Carotenoids convert into vitamin A, stimulate NK cell production and also have anti-inflammatory properties

Organosulphides stimulate macrophage and lymphocyte action

EFAs, most notably omega-6, help red blood cells keep their shape, and so support discocytes and discourage non-discocytes, which are the less effective red blood cells

Probiotics stimulate immune response in the gastrointestinal tract, and also help produce vitamin K, which is required for blood clotting

✔ Friends	*foods to go for*	✘ Foes	*foods to avoid*
Protein, fat Zinc Iron	Eggs, liver, cheese, apricots, sweet potato, butternut squash, peppers (especially red and orange)	Plant sterols Low-fat diets	• **Phytates,** such as cereal grains, legumes like chickpeas, beans and lentils, and plant tissue (Note: plant tissue includes all vegetables and so the importance of these for fibre and nutrient content has to be considered in relation to their benefit over the antagonistic properties of phytates.) • **Excessive soya products** • **Raw cruciferous vegetables** • **Red rice** • **Millet**
Folic acid Vitamin B12	Chicken, lamb, eggs, avocado, cabbage, cauliflower, legumes and brown rice	Overcooking or freezing	
Some evidence that bioflavonoids aid its absorption	Limes, lemons, sweet potatoes, berries, peppers, cauliflower, kale, soft fruits	Excessive water intake	
Vitamin C Selenium	Avocados, almonds, peanuts, sunflower seeds, olive oil, eggs, tuna	Low-fat diets Plant sterols	
Vitamin B6 Protein	Seafood, chicken, oats, brown rice, pumpkin seeds	Excess cellulose & phytates High calcium intake Alcohol & refined sugar	
Iodine	Liver, halibut, cod, tuna, salmon, prawns, mushrooms, sole, mackerel, onions, Brazil nuts, sesame seeds, cashew nuts, kidney beans	Low intake of copper and iron	
Selenium	Seaweeds, kelp, seafood and garlic	Soya, raw cruciferous vegetables, red rice, millet and cassava	
	Citrus fruits, green and white tea, red wine, dark chocolate	Dehydration	
	Carrots, pumpkins, sweet potatoes, tomatoes, watermelon, dark leafy greens, blackcurrants, potatoes, mangoes, red peppers	Artificial fats	
Probiotics	Garlic, onions, chives, shallots and leeks	Microwave cooking	
Selenium Vitamins C, E, B3, B6, carotene zinc, magnesium	Walnuts, sesame seeds, pumpkin seeds, almonds and their oils	Overheating Saturated fats	
	Kefir, sauerkraut, yoghurt and miso; functional foods containing probiotics; tomatoes, onions, garlic and bananas for the oligosaccharides	Refined sugar, alcohol Excess yeast in foods	

Dealing
with stress

STRESS IS EVERYWHERE IT SEEMS, and it's always seen as a bad thing, as it is often associated with being unable to cope, or feeling that there are too many demands being made of us. In fact, stress actually refers to any stimulus that changes the way we react, think or feel. These stimuli are varied, and the modern world has added so many new anxieties that lots of us are in a state of stress every waking hour.

Let's take a look what physiological changes occur when we are stressed. It's worth remembering that as human beings we are rather cleverly designed. Originally, the response to stress was needed to provide us with the ability to hunt for food and also to avoid danger. This reaction, the 'fight or flight' response as it is known, causes many changes that enhance performance and ability. The response occurs mainly in the adrenal glands, but the liver and thyroid gland also respond to the stress stimulus as well.

On sensing stress, the adrenal glands produce both adrenaline and nor-adrenaline. Together these affect several other areas of the body, all in preparation for an increase in available energy that would have been needed to fight our prey or escape while increasing overall alertness and preparing for potential injury. The fight or flight mechanism will:

• Raise the heart rate and the force of each heartbeat.
• Retain fluids.
• Increase blood pressure.

- Dilate blood vessels in the brain, muscles and heart.
- Constrict blood vessels in the skin and spleen.
- Convert glucose stored as glycogen back into glucose.

These processes increase energy levels in another way too, as they divert energy away from areas that are not especially important for the potential battle, most notably digestion.

When the stress of day-to-day life was limited to extremes of temperature, hunting for food and self-preservation, the stress response would have been invoked when required. Once the stress had passed, the body would have returned to a state of relative relaxation. The modern world is such that, as sources of stress are now often unremitting – if you bear in mind that anything that triggers the stress response leads to physiological changes, then how many of us are in a state of high anxiety induced by constantly raised levels of adrenaline?

Remember that stress is caused by anything that you personally find stressful, be that daily situations, such as traffic or emails, or things that sit in the back of your mind causing long-term anxiety, such as finances or family issues. So it follows that our modern lives are full of potential stressors, and that's just those that come from the outside world. Internal sources of stress include blood glucose imbalances, poor sleep quality and general fatigue, all of which can trigger adrenaline to be increased.

In the short term, the stress response gives us energy and allows us to apply ourselves to the task at hand. However, we have an inbuilt ability to cope with levels of stress, and if they are surpassed, then the stress response can lead to health issues that often result in illness or altered behaviour. The sheer amount of potential stressors that we face in a day means that it's possible to spend much of it running on adrenaline. This may be exciting and exhilarating for some, but it's like sitting in a car with your foot pressing down the accelerator pedal, yet the car is in neutral or park, and the handbrake is on. The energy produced by adrenaline is simply not needed, and has a detrimental effect on our health, as it taxes the 'engine', that is us.

Symptoms of not coping with stress include irritable bowel syndrome (IBS) and other digestive problems, as energy is diverted away from digestion, leading to poor absorption. Blood pressure increases, and can remain elevated while the blood becomes thicker (in preparation for injury), leading to cardiovascular complications. Water is retained and weight gain is common, as glucose levels are disrupted. As a result we might try some diet to lose weight, causing further stress. It's also common to have interrupted sleep during times of extreme stress, and this leads to reliance on caffeine and sugars for energy, which in turn lead to other issues. For example, male baldness is linked to stress as excess stress hormones, cortisol for example, interrupt levels of testosterone, and so sexual appetite and performance can be affected, which has a detrimental influence on relationships. The immune system is also impaired by excess stress hormones as they inhibit the action of the white blood cells (see pages 108–9).

You can see all too well what constant stress can do to the body, but there are several steps that can be taken to alleviate the ill-effects of stress. Obviously, reducing the stress itself would be a good start, but I accept that this may not be possible. In fact, when we are feeling stressed even small issues that would normally not cause any anxiety can become a source of irritation, and so working out what matters a lot and what matters less is important. Other steps to consider are massage, acupuncture, yoga, Pilates or any hobby that offers relief and distraction.

Obviously, what we choose to eat is going to make a difference as to how well we handle stress, and to reduce the ill-effects of long-term stress. The rush of energy that increased adrenaline levels supply is not without cost. In order to get that burst, metabolism of fats, proteins and carbohydrates is speeded up. In doing so, both phosphorus and potassium are excreted more quickly. Magnesium is also depleted as the adrenal glands are significant users of the mineral along with vitamins B5 and C.

Nutrients for combating stress

To counteract the thickened state of the blood caused by the 'fight or flight' response, Essential Fatty Acids and vitamin E would be useful, perhaps best if they are found together rather than concentrating on vitamin E intake in isolation.

nutrients and their role

Phosphorus as levels of this mineral are depleted when metabolic processes speed up in times of stress, due to it being a major component of ATP (the usable form of energy)

Potassium is required for the metabolism of proteins and various enzymes that contribute to the formation of energy from glucose

Vitamin C is required for adrenal function as it is utilized in the formation of adrenaline and cortisol

Vitamin B5 is used to make stress hormones and thus the requirement takes on added importance in times of stress

Magnesium is required for adrenal gland function, especially for the formation of adrenaline

Essential fatty acids with inherent vitamin E, as in times of stress the immune system becomes impaired, and inflammation is more likely. Additionally, the blood thickens when we are under stress and essential fats can counteract this, which reduces the risk of cardiovascular complications

A day's Supereating

BREAKFAST
small smoothie made from citrus fruits, melon, strawberries and blackcurrants, with some pumpkin seeds and a spoonful of plain yoghurt

MORNING SNACK
avocado dip made with lemon juice and diced tomato, and eaten with sliced raw red and orange peppers

LUNCH
baked potato with chickpeas and salad made with salad leaves and a choice of any dark green leafy vegetable, such as spinach and broccoli, and sun-dried tomato

AFTERNOON SNACK
chopped shelled hard-boiled eggs with cucumber slices

DINNER
flaked salmon stir-fry, made with sweet potato, quinoa, bok choi and spinach, topped with sunflower seeds

✔ Friends	*foods to go for*	✘ Foes	*foods to avoid*
Vitamin D	Seafoods particularly roes; meat particularly liver; eggs and dairy foods; pulses, quinoa; nuts and seeds	High intake of fructose (fruit sugars)	• **Overcooked foods** (steam vegetables lightly) • **Red meat and dairy products** contain saturated fats and should be minimized, to perhaps twice a week of each • **Raw eggs** • **Salt** (use herbs or lemon juice to enhance the flavour of food) • **Licorice** • Limit **fruit** to 2 pieces a day and increase vegetable intake to compensate • **Concentrated fruit juices**
None	Avocados, tomatoes, tomato paste, sun-dried tomatoes and dried fruit; potatoes, sweet potatoes, squash, cucumbers, peppers, banana, apricots and dark green vegetables (but see Foods to Avoid)	Over-exercise (itself a potential stressor) Diarrhoea Licorice Salt	
None	All fresh fruit and vegetables, but particularly good sources include acerola cherries, all citrus fruits, cantaloupe melons, pineapples, blackcurrants, strawberries, peppers, potatoes and dark green leafy vegetables, such as kale (but see Foods to Avoid)	Cooking Infections Excess hydration as the vitamin is water-borne and easily excreted	
Vitamin C Biotin Other B vitamins	Vitamin B5 is found in all foods, but particularly good sources are liver and kidneys. Poultry and red meat are good sources, and dairy foods, particularly yoghurt, contain high levels, while avocados are excellent sources (but see Foods to Avoid). Of the pulses, lentils provide the highest levels. Tomato concentrate in paste and purée also provides good levels, as do potatoes and sweet potato. Sunflower seeds are also a rich source	Freezing and processing of food Impaired digestion	
Calcium Vitamin D	Oat bran, brown rice, quinoa, pumpkin and sunflower seeds, whole grains, nuts, lentils and dark green leafy vegetables (so vegetarians will find it easy to obtain optimum levels)	Phosphoric acid (carbonated drinks) Oxalic acid (in soft fruits, quinoa, nuts, berries and beans) Low calcium intake Processed grains	
Vitamin E (always found alongside EFAs in food) Vitamins B3, B6 and C together with magnesium help fats become anti-inflammatory	Fish, nuts, avocado, seeds and their oils	Overheating of foods Saturated fats	

Improving
digestive health

WHEN WE TALK ABOUT DIGESTION we should be aware that this general term covers three areas – the breakdown of food, the absorption of the nutrients contained within it and the elimination of the waste by-product.

Obviously we are all familiar with the process of eating, but in order to apply the Supereating template to digestion, we need to understand a little more about what's involved. The process of digestion starts with chewing, during which the food is mixed with saliva, which itself contains several enzymes that also break down the food. Saliva is mostly water, and this helps moisten the food for several reasons, not least to avoid choking. The importance of chewing food well does seem to be rather overlooked when it comes to eating – I believe that so many of us eat far too quickly, and expect the digestive system to do the job for us.

Once the food is in a comfortable state to be swallowed, it drops down into the stomach through a valve. In the stomach, gastric acid starts its work in further breaking down the food. This acid is powerful stuff as it consists largely

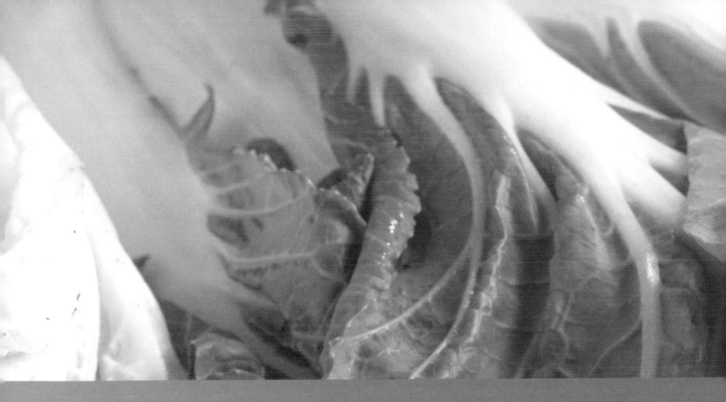

of hydrochloric acid, with some sodium and potassium chloride mixed in too. The tissue and structure of the stomach are protected from the potentially harmful effects of the acid by thick layers of mucous. The acid is actually made by cells in the stomach called parietal cells. Bear in mind that bacteria and pathogens are mostly destroyed by this highly acidic environment, and so the gastric acid also forms part of the immune system.

The stomach also produces some digestive enzymes that contribute to the breakdown of foods, notably intrinsic factor, a substance that also comes from the parietal cells and enables vitamin B12 to be absorbed, a lack of which is associated with anaemia.

Once the stomach acid has done its job, the food is now in the form of a gel-like liquid known as chyme. Carbohydrates, especially simple ones that have few bonds to hold them together, tend to pass through the stomach quite swiftly. Complex carbohydrates by comparison, take longer, with fat and protein being the last to pass through as they are harder to break down.

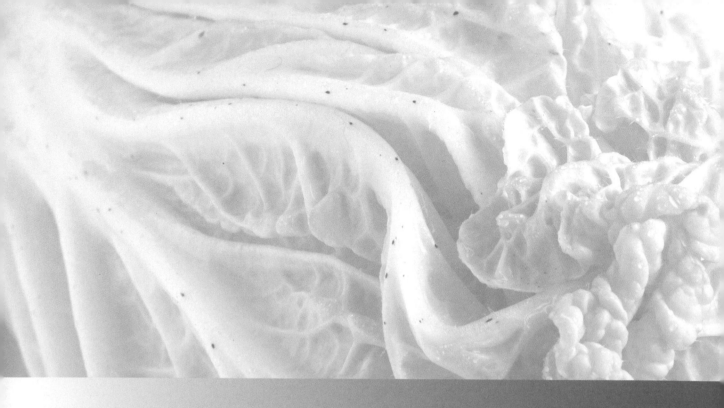

This newly formed chyme is pushed along the digestive system by involuntary muscle (peristaltic) movement, during which time it is exposed to the multitude of absorption sites. The surface of the small intestine, where the majority of absorption takes place, is covered in finger-like protrusions through which nutrients are absorbed and then passed through membranes to reach the blood, where they are transported into cells that use them for a wide variety of functions. Waste products are added to the remaining chyme (including excess cholesterol and broken-down red blood cells) before it is passed out of the body and ends up in your bathroom.

The whole digestive system is a highly complicated process, and it is quite common to have poor digestion, which can result in many of the day-to-day health issues that don't quite constitute an illness, but do cause discomfort and less than optimal functioning. These might include bloating, gas, belching and irregular bowel movements. Obviously there are several reasons why anyone might experience these from time to time, but the chances are increased given the stress of modern life, the sort of food we tend to choose (refined sugars, excess carbohydrates and alcohol, for example) and the pace at which we eat it.

Nutrients for the various stages of digestion

Like all the workings of the body, every single nutrient is used in most processes. No one nutrient does one thing, but instead adds to the total mix. Therefore it is not easy to identify which nutrients are most important, but if we look more closely at the three stages of digestion – breakdown, absorption and elimination – then it becomes easier to highlight the key nutrients.

Breakdown

It is a fact that the breakdown of food relies mainly on chewing. It may seem mundane, but I have worked with many clients over the years who have benefited from improved digestive health by remembering to chew their food more. Time-consuming and routine it may be, but it is a worthwhile investment. Also, as saliva consists of 98% water, adequate hydration is vital.

Aside from chewing, gastric acid is obviously important in the breakdown, and the parietal cells require zinc and vitamin B6 to function well. Additionally, as the parietal cells that create it work at an increased rate compared to many other cells, they require more oxygen, and thus iron levels should be optimized.

Absorption

Absorption of nutrients relies on several factors, not least the efficient movement of the chyme as it passes through the digestive system. This peristaltic movement relies on muscle contraction – the muscles behind the lump of chyme contract whilst those just ahead of it relax, squeezing it along and exposing it to as many absorption sites as possible. Efficient muscle contraction and relaxation is linked to sufficient levels of magnesium and calcium.

Absorption is also linked to levels of probiotics, and so the factors that influence their concentration are very relevant.

Elimination

Once again, muscle contraction is important and so magnesium and calcium are important. Fibre is also important as it helps bulk up the stool, and helps remove excess cholesterol from the gastrointestinal (GI) tract, preventing it from being reabsorbed. Water is also a vital component to help moisten the stool for ease of passing.

Nutrients for digestive health

In addition to helping break down foods, probiotics help maintain the overall health of the lining of the digestive system, protecting it from pathogens that can occupy absorption sites. Probiotics also help the movement of food along the gastrointestinal (GI) tract.

Note: hard water can reduce calcium absorption, so if you know that you live in a hard water area, use a softener when steaming vegetables.

A day's Supereating

BREAKFAST
oat bran with soya milk or skimmed cows' milk, with mixed nuts and seeds, especially sunflower seeds and hazelnuts, topped with sliced banana

MORNING SNACK
dried apricots in a little plain yoghurt

LUNCH
grilled fresh sardines, tinned sardines or salmon, served in a salad made with mixed salad leaves

AFTERNOON SNACK
hummus on a rye cracker

DINNER
grilled seafood or roast chicken served with lentils, broccoli, peas and chard

nutrients and their role

Magnesium is required alongside calcium as these are the major contributing nutrients in peristaltic movement. One tell-tale sign of low magnesium levels is constipation and I often find that increasing magnesium levels makes a significant difference

Calcium is required for the contraction of muscles and is thus important for peristaltic movement, making digestion and elimination more efficient

Probiotics are partially responsible for digestion, as they actually continue to break down food particles when they enter the large intestine

Iron is required for haemoglobin, which carries oxygen to the hard-working parietal cells

Vitamin B6 is required for the parietal cells

Zinc is required by the parietal cells in the tissue that lines the stomach

✔ Friends	*foods to go for*	✘ Foes	*foods to avoid*
Calcium Vitamin D	Oat bran, brown rice, quinoa, pumpkin and sunflower seeds, whole grains, nuts, lentils and dark green leafy vegetables (but see Foods to Avoid)	Phosphoric acid (in carbonated drinks) Oxalic acid (soft fruits, quinoa, nuts and beans)	• **Carbonated drinks** • **Raw vegetables**, so eat steamed instead • **Alcohol** • **Vinegar**, including balsamic • **Excess tea and coffee**, limit to one of each daily • **Refined sugar** • **Grains** can be limited but not avoided altogether to manage phytate intake
Vitamin D Magnesium Potassium (reduces calcium excretion) Probiotics (increase calcium absorption from some dairy foods) Inulin (in garlic, asparagus, etc.)	Best sources are soft fish bones, so eat whitebait, sardines and tinned salmon (also natural sources of vitamin D to enhance absorption). Vegetarian sources are fermented dairy products, like live yoghurt and cottage cheese. Fortified soya yoghurt and tofu supply easily absorbable calcium. Cheddar cheese is high in calcium, but eat in moderation as high in saturated fats. Good levels in Chinese lettuce, bok choi, kale, broccoli, almonds and sesame seeds	Oxalic acid (see magnesium) Phytates (in most grains) Low hydrochloric acid in the stomach Coffee Salt Phosphoric acid (in carbonated drinks) Refined sugar	
Inulin (acts a prebiotic) Oligosaccharides	Kefir, sauerkraut, yoghurt and miso; functional foods containing probiotics; tomatoes, onions, garlic and bananas for the oligosaccharides	Antibiotics, alcohol	
Citric acid Tartaric acid Malic acid Vitamin C Lactic acid Amino acids, most notably cysteine	Liver, beef, lamb and venison; good vegetarian sources include chickpeas, beans and peas (but see Foods to Avoid), chard and spinach, dried apricots and tomato paste; citrus fruits for the citric acid, grapes for the malic acid, fermented foods such as yoghurt for the lactic acid, poultry, yoghurt, garlic, onions, wheatgerm, Brussels sprouts and broccoli for the cysteine	Tannins (tea, coffee, etc.) Polyphenols (in red wine) Legumes, fruits and vegetables (inappropriate to avoid, so go for friends) Phosphoric acid (in carbonated drinks) Excessive zinc and/or calcium supplementation	
Folic acid Vitamin B12 (B6 is required to help release B12 and B3 metabolism has to be good to make B6 available)	Poultry, red meat and offal (particularly liver); pulses (particularly chickpeas); fish; green vegetables (particularly spinach), asparagus, avocados, cauliflowers, peppers and chestnut mushrooms; root vegetables, leeks and onions; bananas and cantaloupe; cooking with turmeric and ginger could also improve levels	Cooking and, especially, freezing food High levels of acid (i.e. vinegar or the like) during cooking	
Vitamin B6 Cysteine, an amino acid found in protein foods	Adequate zinc in soil is necessary for plant uptake, so good sources depend on locale; the most available form comes from protein, like meat, game, liver, eggs and seafood (particularly oysters); cheese, yoghurt, beans, nuts and seeds are good sources, but the zinc is less absorbable	Phytates, mainly in grains Cellulose, in leafy plants, so less raw veg (steam) Excess intake of calcium, copper or phosphorus Alcohol and refined sugar	

Eating for
greater energy

FEELING UNUSUALLY TIRED isn't uncommon, and in today's pressurized environment, it's an accepted part of life for many people. While a large number of people may be overly stressed or sleep-deprived, I am confident that improving diet can make a difference.

We eat for a variety of reasons, ranging from hunger to social conditioning. Simple hunger is a signal that we need fuel and so, from a purely physiological point of view, this is a sign that we are about to require fuel to make energy. Therefore all eating is actually done to create energy, in addition to facilitating the repair and renewal of the body.

All nutrients are required to make energy, but the process of making the sort of energy that we think of needing for things like moving, running, etc., is done in the cells, and in this process some nutrients have a more pivotal role to play than others. There are few, if any, minerals, vitamins, amino acids and essential fats that are not used in the process of creating energy, and so isolating those that are more important than others is not an easy process. Those that I feel are most relevant have been chosen to demonstrate how the Supereating approach can be used to enhance energy levels.

Bear in mind that the process of making energy is highly complex and evolved, and the scale of the various components is far smaller than most people can imagine. For example, in a cell we might find 2,000 areas that make energy, together with a billion energy units. Therefore, the explanation given here is a very simplified and basic one.

What we eat and drink is broken down by the digestive system (see pages 118–123), the nutrients and glucose are released and are then filtered through membranes into the bloodstream before entering the cells in various forms. In every cell are something called mitochondria (cells have anywhere between 500 and 2,000 of them). In our simplified version it's easier to imagine these as an extraordinary power station – glucose is converted into pyruvic acid that is delivered to the power station which, in turn, uses it to create power. It's not just glucose that is required, but other substances that are derived from food such as amino acids and fats too. Glucose comes mainly from carbohydrates, while amino acids are found in protein and, lastly, fats are used too.

All food groups are broken down in the digestive system and the end-products are separated into their constituent parts, which are then also delivered into a part of the mitochondria, or 'power station' in our simple version, known as the Krebs Cycle (also sometimes called the citric acid cycle). Bear in mind that any one cell might have 2,000 mitochondria, so the parts involved are infinitesimal.

Within the mitochondria there occurs a complex and intricate process in which pyruvic acid, glucose, amino acids and the end product of fats are oxidized and converted into adenosine 5'-triphosphate, or ATP as it is known. This is the form of energy that is then used throughout the body. Just to give you an idea of how involved the process is, it is estimated that a typical cell contains a billion molecules of ATP, each of which lives for less than a minute. ATP is the form of energy that powers most of the bodily functions.

Nutrients for boosting energy

There are several substances that are part of the Krebs Cycle, and thus many nutrients are involved in making energy. However, there are some that are involved in more than one section, and it is these that are the focus of our Supereating approach. Concentrating on these nutrients can have a noticeable effect on energy levels for those of us that are flagging and not feeling quite as energetic as usual.

A day's Supereating

BREAKFAST
mixed grain porridge made using soya or skimmed milk, topped with flaked almonds and chopped strawberries

MORNING SNACK
fruit salad made with oranges, grapefruit and cherries

LUNCH
grilled fresh tuna or tinned tuna with salad leaves, peppers, carrots and tomato, with a dressing of lemon juice and olive oil

AFTERNOON SNACK
hard-boiled egg, chopped and made into a paste with plain yoghurt, avocado and black pepper, spread on oatcakes

DINNER
stir-fry of chard, kale, spinach, broccoli, mushrooms and peppers, mixed with quinoa and served with either grilled calves' liver, steak or lamb fillet

nutrients and their role

Probiotics help the creation of B vitamins from other foods, but also make a small amount themselves. They also help release magnesium from food

Magnesium acts as a glucose carrier, working to transport glucose to the cells where it is absorbed ready for conversion to pyruvic acid and on to the Krebs Cycle

Chromium makes insulin more potent

Vitamin B1 has a direct role to play in the conversion of glucose into pyruvic acid, as well as in the creation of ATP in the Krebs Cycle. It is also used to turn fats into pyruvic acid, thus helping in the process of creating energy from the fat we eat

Vitamin B2, like B1, helps in the creation of pyruvic acid and is used to convert fats into ATP as well as in the Krebs Cycle. B2 is also required to move electrons around, so that energy is released from the cycle

Vitamin B3 is required in the Krebs Cycle in addition to helping in the process of fats becoming pyruvic acid. Lastly, it is required to help carry electrons out of the Krebs cycle, which is the last stage of creating ATP

Vitamin C is an essential part of the creation of ATP in the Krebs cycle and also in the last stage of energy release, called the electron transfer chain

Biotin helps amino acids in proteins become pyruvic acid, and also in getting into the Krebs cycle. It is also required in the breakdown of fats into energy

✔ Friends	*foods to go for*	✘ Foes	*foods to avoid*
Inulin (acts a prebiotic) Oligosaccharides	Kefir, sauerkraut, yoghurt and miso; functional foods containing probiotics; tomatoes, onions, garlic and bananas for the oligosaccharides	Antibiotics Alcohol	• **Carbonated drinks** • **Excessive tea and coffee**, one cup of each daily is the maximum • **Raw egg** • **Low protein intake** • **Almonds** • **Peanuts** • **Alcohol** should be minimized
Calcium Vitamin D	Excellent food sources include oat bran, brown rice, quinoa, pumpkin and sunflower seeds, whole grains, nuts, lentils and dark green leafy vegetables (so vegetarians will find it easy to obtain optimum levels)	Phosphoric acid (in carbonated drinks) Oxalic acid (in soft fruits, quinoa, nuts, berries and beans)	
Adequate levels of vitamin B3 and glutathione are needed to make the active form of chromium, GTF	Liver, poultry, shellfish, broccoli, brewer's yeast, whole grains, pulses and spices, grape juice	Refined foods high in sugar and carbohydrates increase demand Trauma and mental stress increase excretion Calcium carbonate (hard water) and phytic acid (coffee, whole grains and legumes) lower absorption	
Other B vitamins Probiotics Magnesium	Whole grains, lentils and beans provide reasonable levels of Vitamin B1, but the highest levels can be found in a serving of wheat germ, sunflower seeds and lean pork	Alcohol, processed foods, excess tea and coffee, raw fish, overcooking	
Vitamin B1 in moderate amounts Other B vitamins Probiotics	Dairy, particularly yoghurt; eggs; fish (especially trout and tuna); broccoli, spinach and avocados; red meat and dark chicken meat; grains, particularly oat bran, wheat germ, quinoa and rye	Stress Alcohol Exposure to light	
Vitamin B6 and iron help release B3 from tryptophan Other B vitamins	High-protein foods, such as poultry, fish, red meat and liver; chestnut mushrooms; foods high in tryptophan will help boost niacin levels, so dairy foods and eggs would be good choices	Low-protein diets, as amino acids are required to help release B3 Overcooking	
Bioflavonoids	All fresh fruit and vegetables, but particularly good sources include acerola cherries, all citrus fruits, cantaloupe melons, pineapples, blackcurrants, strawberries, peppers, potatoes and dark green leafy vegetables such as kale	Excessive liquid intake as the vitamin is water-soluble Cooking	
Probiotics Other B vitamins, notably B5	Offal (particularly liver); fish, egg yolk and soya products; nuts (notably hazelnuts); Swiss chard, sweet potato, tomatoes, carrots and avocados	Poor digestion Raw egg white Processed foods	

Maintaining
heart health

PART OF ANY HEALTHY LIFESTYLE has to involve looking after both the heart and the cardiovascular system, and a good diet together with regular exercise can help reduce the risk of disease in these areas. A lot has been written about the best diet for heart health, yet applying the Supereating approach can make an appropriate diet that little bit more effective. There are several areas on which to focus when we think of a diet beneficial to the heart:

BLOOD PRESSURE

The heart itself is actually a muscle that drives blood around the veins and arteries. The internal surface of these 'tubes' can be eroded, and when damage is noted, the body will repair the area by applying smooth muscle cells to it, much like plaster on a wound.

The area of repair is not identical to the original lining, however, and is effectively a little sticky, thereby attracting elements contained in the blood to it, including cholesterol, proteins, calcium and lipids, collectively referred to as plaque. If the repaired areas repeatedly attract such elements, then, quite simply, they grow and intrude upon the unobstructed passing of the blood through these 'tubes', decreasing their internal circumference. Inevitably, this effect, known as atherosclerosis, increases blood pressure, and if a repaired area gets dislodged and detaches, which is more likely as the blood rushes past the obstruction at a higher speed, this can lead to a blockage, resulting in a heart attack or stroke.

FREE RADICALS AND ANTIOXIDANTS

Many people are familiar with the term 'antioxidant' as it is often mentioned when talking about the benefits of fruits, vegetables, red wine and chocolate. Antioxidants do as their name suggests, they reduce the damaging oxidization of cells that results from contact with free radicals. Free radicals are substances that are the natural by-product of the metabolism, and they result in a single molecule of oxygen being free, allowing it to join other molecules, changing their chemical structure.

Some elements of the cells are more vulnerable to this oxidization effect and the damage that is caused to them by it is a contributing factor in the ageing process. In relation to heart health, free radicals are involved in the process of atherosclerosis.

CHOLESTEROL AND FATS

There are two types of cholesterol, high density lipoprotein and low density lipoprotein, or HDL and LDL as they are more commonly known. There is still some confusion in many people's minds about cholesterol and, in consultations, I find that many people concentrate on lowering cholesterol scores without acknowledging the importance of the other aspects of a healthy diet for the heart. There are a number of points to understand about cholesterol, the most basic being that it is not always a bad thing, as it is required for some basic bodily functions. Cholesterol is an oily substance and doesn't travel in blood easily, and so is wrapped in a type of fat called a lipoprotein, which is essentially a method of transporting substances around the body. Of the two types of cholesterol, HDL and LDL, it's the latter that we need to keep an eye on, as it is this type that delivers substances to where they are required, whilst the HDL removes the excess (a very easy way to remember which is the 'good' cholesterol is simply to remember that the 'h' is for 'happy' or 'helpful').

Cholesterol comes from two sources, the liver and the diet. The liver makes some 80% of total levels with the rest coming from the diet. Cholesterol is found in some foods, such as eggs, offal and dairy products, but intake of saturated fats will also result in increased cholesterol levels, even though the fats don't contain any, as the process of breaking down saturated fats results in cholesterol being produced. To reduce the risk of cardiovascular disease linked to increased levels of cholesterol the Supereating approach takes into account both the creation of cholesterol and also its dismantling and removal from the body.

HOMOCYSTEINE

Homocysteine may not be that familiar to you, but it is as important to heart health as cholesterol, yet has not received anywhere near the level of attention. Homocysteine can be derived from methionine, an amino acid found in protein foods (but this does not mean that proteins should be avoided at all) considered essential for growth and repair of the body. Excess homocysteine interferes with enzymes that, in turn, will affect both elastin and collagen, and is considered to be toxic as it corrodes the structure of arteries. Homocysteine levels can build up if there are deficiencies of specific nutrients (vitamins B6, folic acid and B12). Although research indicates that taking supplementation of these nutrients not deficient doesn't alter homocysteine levels, Supereating can help derive more of these important nutrients from the diet to avoid deficiencies.

Nutrients for heart health

Several nutrients have antioxidant properties, but a number have more established roles in the reduction of risks from heart disease.

nutrients and their role

Calcium is required for the action of the heart muscle and also for its role in reducing blood pressure

Magnesium is involved in the relaxation of the heart muscle and also required to help control blood pressure

Potassium levels are affected when sodium intake is too high. To counteract raised blood pressure a low-salt diet combined with plenty of potassium-rich foods is recommended

Essential fatty acids are required to help thin the blood, partly due to their vitamin E content (vitamin E occurs naturally in foods containing EFAs because it works to protect these susceptible fats, see pages 90–91)

Folic acid is required to reduce levels of homocysteine

Vitamin B6 is required to reduce levels of homocysteine

(table continued overleaf)

A day's Supereating

BREAKFAST
oat porridge made with unsweetened soya milk or skimmed cows' milk, topped with blueberries and sunflower seeds

MORNING SNACK
an apple or pear with 5 cashew nuts

LUNCH
grilled fresh sardines or tinned sardines, served with bok choi, cooked lentils, salad leaves and sun-dried tomatoes

AFTERNOON SNACK
half a small avocado

DINNER
miso soup with shredded ginger, followed by grilled chicken breast, served with brown rice, asparagus and peppers; with a dressing made from tomato paste, crushed garlic and plain yoghurt

✔ Friends	*foods to go for*	✘ Foes	*foods to avoid*
Vitamin D Magnesium, Potassium reduces excretion Probiotics increase absorption from some dairy foods Inulin, found in asparagus, garlic	Best sources are soft fish bones, so eat whitebait, sardines and tinned salmon (also natural sources of vitamin D) to enhance absorption. Vegetarian sources are fermented dairy products, like live yoghurt and cottage cheese. Fortified soya yoghurt and tofu supply easily absorbable calcium. Cheddar cheese is high in calcium, but eat in moderation as high in saturated fats. Good levels in Chinese lettuce, bok choi, kale, broccoli, almonds and sesame seeds	Oxalic acid (in soft fruits, quinoa, nuts and beans) Phytates (in most grains) Low hydrochloric acid in the stomach Coffee Salt Phosphoric acid (in carbonated drinks) Refined sugar	• **Low-fat diets** • **Alcohol** • **Refined sugar** • **Phytates**: limit grain intake to manage levels • **Raw vegetables** (steamed is preferable) • **Artificial fats**
Calcium Vitamin D	Oat bran, brown rice, quinoa, pumpkin and sunflower seeds; whole grains, nuts, lentils, dark green leafy vegetables (but see Foods to Avoid)	Phosphoric acid (in carbonated drinks) Oxalic acid (see above)	
None	Avocados, tomatoes, tomato paste, sun-dried tomatoes and dried fruit; potatoes, sweet potatoes, squash, cucumbers, peppers, banana, apricots and dark green vegetables	Diarrhoea Over-exercise Licorice	
Vitamins B3, B6 and C, magnesium and zinc all help EFA utilization Vitamin E, carotene and selenium protect the fats from free radical damage	Nuts, seeds, fish, avocado and oils	Trans and saturated fats block absorption while bright lights or high temperatures can denature the fats	
Thiamine, riboflavin, niacin, B6 and B12 all aid utilization	Green vegetables, especially Cos lettuce, avocado, asparagus, spinach and broccoli; even better sources are pulses, particularly lentils; liver provides the highest levels of folic acid	Alcohol, overcooking vegetables, and low B6 and B12 can all suppress folic acid function	
Folic acid Vitamin B12 (B6 is required to help release B12) Vitamin B3 metabolism has to be good to make B6 available	Poultry, red meat and offal (particularly liver); pulses (particularly chickpeas); fish; green vegetables (particularly spinach), asparagus, avocados, cauliflowers, peppers and chestnut mushrooms; root vegetables, leeks and onions; bananas and cantaloupe; cooking with turmeric and ginger could also improve levels	Cooking and, especially, freezing food High levels of acid during cooking, i.e. with vinegar or the like	*(table continued overleaf)*

Nutrients for heart health (continued)

nutrients and their role

Vitamin B12 is required to reduce levels of homocysteine

Probiotics help in the excretion of cholesterol

Chromium helps reduce cholesterol and improves the levels of HDL (good) cholesterol

Organosulphides are phytochemicals found mainly in garlic which can have a positive effect on reducing blood pressure and also have cholesterol-lowering properties

Vitamin C is often thought of as 'the' nutrient for heart health, and has several roles to play: it can help reduce cholesterol, acts as an antioxidant and helps convert fats into energy (unconverted they can build up in the blood, increasing the risk of atherosclerosis

Betacarotene and carotenoids are noted for their antioxidant properties

Zinc is noted for its antioxidant properties

✔ Friends	*foods to go for*	✘ Foes	*foods to avoid*
Other B vitamins	Red meat, particularly liver, poultry and game; oily fish; eggs and dairy food; fermented foods, such as yoghurt	Poor digestion Anaemia Vegan diet	see page 133
Inulin (acts a prebiotic) Oligosaccharides	Kefir, sauerkraut, yoghurt and miso; functional foods containing probiotics; tomatoes, onions, garlic and bananas for the oligosaccharides	Antibiotics Alcohol	
Vitamin B3 Glutathione	Liver, poultry, shellfish, broccoli, brewer's yeast, whole grains, pulses and spices, grape juice	Excessive sugar intake Low-protein diets (they increase demand) Phytates (in most grains) Hard water (containing calcium carbonate)	
Crushing garlic makes it more potent	Garlic, onion, shallots, leeks, chives	Microwave cooking	
	All fresh fruit and vegetables, but particularly good sources include acerola cherries, all citrus fruits, cantaloupe melons, pineapples, blackcurrants, strawberries, peppers, potatoes and dark green leafy vegetables, such as kale	Excessive liquid intake as the vitamin is water-soluble Cooking	
	Carrots, sweet potato, spinach, kale, peaches and apricots provide beta-carotene; carrots, pumpkins and red and yellow peppers provide alpha-carotene; pumpkin, red peppers and orange-coloured fruit provide cryptoxanthin; tomatoes, particularly processed, as in paste or tinned, are the best source of lycopene; leafy greens, such as kale and spinach as well as peas and corn, provide lutein and zeaxanthin; salmon, prawns and other seafood are a good source of astaxanthin	Low-fat diets Artificial fats	
Vitamin B6 Cysteine, an amino acid found in protein foods	Adequate zinc in soil is necessary for plant uptake, so good sources depend on locale; the most available form comes from protein, like meat, game, liver, eggs and seafood (particularly oysters); cheese, yoghurt, beans, nuts and seeds are good sources, but the zinc is less absorbable	Phytates, mainly in grains Cellulose, in leafy plants, so less raw veg (steam) Excess intake of calcium, copper or phosphorus Alcohol and refined sugar	

Maintaining
general skin health

HAVING 'GOOD' SKIN **is something that we hear a lot about, usually in relation to cosmetics or lotions that promise to add moisture, smooth out wrinkles and lines, cover blemishes and generally contribute to making us feel better about how we look. Obviously it's not just the skin on our faces that we want to look and feel good, but beauty and vanity aside, many people have skin problems, such as rashes, acne, oily or dry skin, and more serious issues ranging from rosacea to psoriasis. The good news is that what you eat can make a significant difference to your overall skin health, and with Supereating we can take that one stage further.**

Much of what we think about when we think of our skin is age-related, and for the Supereating approach to ageing, see page 100. The eating plan that is appropriate for anti-ageing will also be of benefit to the skin. However, in this section, we will be looking at the general health of skin, at how it is made and what nutrients contribute to keeping it supple and flexible, while also seeing what we can do to reduce day-to-day skin problems.

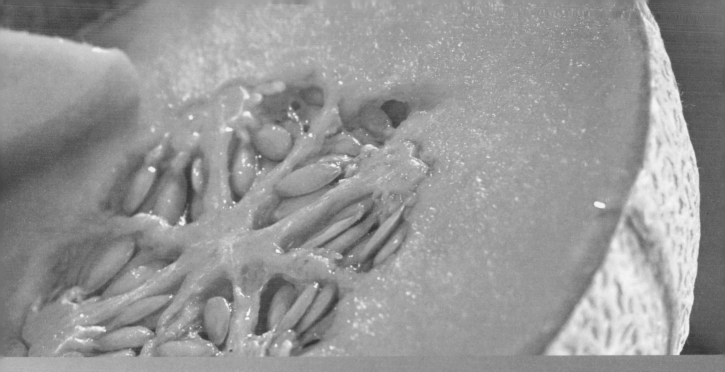

SKIN AND NUTRITION

The skin is the largest organ in the body, and after the liver, is a major route of elimination of toxins and waste. The average adult has skin that covers over 20 square feet and weighs anything up to 13lb (6 kilos). What we think of as skin is actually divided into two parts: the upper, or outer, section, the epidermis, is made up of four or five layers that act as a protection, keeping out microbes and unwanted substances, and repelling water. Skin cells are made deep in the epidermis and are pushed up, layer by layer, until they reach the surface. This process takes around 4 weeks to complete, and so changes in the diet that affect the skin often don't show until this time.

The layer beneath the epidermis, the dermis, is more like connective tissue than the thin layers of skin we are familiar with and it is in this layer that the majority of the skin's collagen is stored. Collagen is a flexible structure made of two amino acids found in proteins, and is dependent on vitamin C for its formation. Without it blood vessels become weak and teeth loose as the collagen is depleted, so a number of skin issues can be directly related to poor levels of vitamin C.

Vitamin C is indeed the most potent nutrient when it comes to skin care, as it also has antioxidant properties, and can combat free radicals which will affect collagen as well as elastin (the flexible tissue that helps skin regain its shape after it is pulled).

Flushing, redness and hives are inflammatory conditions and, if these are your concerns, it is worth looking at the relevant section in the chapter on the immune system, on pages 106–111.

As the skin is an elimination route for toxins, an overworked liver can be linked to skin problems. There are many nutrients that are required for an efficient liver, mainly those with antioxidant properties, as these are directly involved in combining with toxins to render them harmless. Antioxidants are also important for the skin as they offer some protection from the free radical damage that results from normal metabolism, and degraded skin cells will look less than healthy, affecting the appearance of the skin. There is little or no evidence that antioxidants in the diet offer protection from ultraviolet light, but nevertheless they are an important part of a healthy diet for the skin.

The skin cells don't last long and are being constantly replaced, and therefore

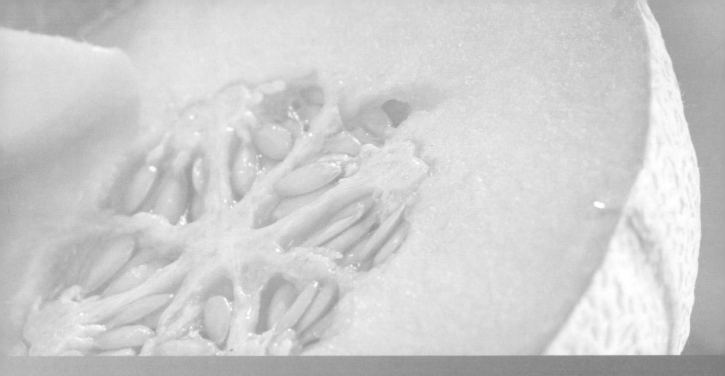

dietary fats are needed as they are important components of every cell, not least skin cells. In order to derive the fats that are required for every cell, biotin is needed and low levels of biotin can quickly result in dry, flaky skin. Biotin comes largely from the diet but some is also made by beneficial bacteria, and so probiotics are also useful for healthy skin. I have found in practice that increasing the levels of probiotics helps many clients with minor skin problems, ranging from acne to dry skin.

Acne is another issue that affects many people, and is linked to several factors, not least sebum production (sebum being the oily substance produced deep in the skin that makes it waterproof). If sebum production is too high, then this will encourage acne or spots – vitamin A can help reduce excess sebum from being produced.

Nutrients for skin health

Vitamin E and essential fats are required to help plump up skin, making it look fresh and dewy, but vitamin E is best consumed with fats as it is always present alongside essential fats in foods, so no special effort is required to find vitamin E.

Zinc is also a vital skin nutrient as it is involved in healing after skin has been damaged, but it also has antioxidant properties.

nutrients and their role

Vitamin A is required for controlling sebum production and for its powers as an antioxidant

Vitamin C for its antioxidant properties and also as it is a major component of collagen

Zinc is noted for its antioxidant properties and role in healing of the skin

Biotin helps derive essential fatty acids from food for use in the skin cells

Probiotics help the creation of B vitamins from other foods, but also make a small amount themselves

Carotenoids such as beta-carotene and others are noted for their antioxidant properties

Essential fatty acids with vitamin E (always found alongside EFAs in food) as in times of stress the immune system becomes impaired, and inflammation is more likely. Additionally, the blood thickens when we are under stress and essential fats can counteract this, which reduces the risk of cardiovascular complications

A day's Supereating

BREAKFAST
smoothie made from plain yoghurt, peach, strawberries and pumpkin seeds

MORNING SNACK
sliced carrots with avocado and tomato salsa dip

LUNCH
omelette with diced squash, red and yellow peppers and peas

AFTERNOON SNACK
sunflower seeds and apricot

DINNER
miso soup, followed by grilled salmon or prawns, served with spinach and a baked sweet potato

✔ Friends	*foods to go for*	✗ Foes	*foods to avoid*
Zinc Iron	The most concentrated source is liver, but eggs, cheese and yoghurt are also good sources; carrots, sweet potato, squash, broccoli, avocado, peaches, apricots, melon, mangoes and papayas are good vegetarian sources	Low level of fat intake Functional foods, especially those that lower cholesterol	• **Low-fat diets** • **Artificial fats,** such as in cholesterol-lowering functional foods • **Raw egg** • **Phytate levels**: grain intake should be limited to manage levels • **Raw vegetables** (steamed is preferable)
	Citrus fruits, kiwi fruit, sweet potato, peppers	Excessive liquid intake as water-soluble Cooking	
Vitamin B6 Cysteine, an amino acid found in protein foods	Adequate zinc in soil is necessary for plant uptake, so good sources depend on locale; the most available form comes from protein, like meat, game, liver, eggs and seafood (particularly oysters); cheese, yoghurt, beans, nuts and seeds are good sources, but the zinc is less absorbable	Phytates, mainly in grains Cellulose, in leafy plants, so less raw veg (steam) Excess intake of calcium, copper or phosphorus Alcohol and refined sugar	
Other B vitamins, notably B5 Probiotics	Organ meat, particularly liver; fish; egg yolk; soya products; nuts, particularly hazelnuts and almonds; vegetables especially Swiss chard, sweet potatoes, tomatoes, carrots and avocados	Poor levels of probiotics Raw eggs reduce biotin levels	
Inulin (acts a prebiotic) Oligosaccharides	Kefir, sauerkraut, yoghurt and miso; functional foods containing probiotics; tomatoes, onions, garlic and bananas for the oligosaccharides	Antibiotics Alcohol	
	Carrots and sweet potato, spinach and kale, peaches and apricots provide beta-carotene; carrots, pumpkins and red and yellow peppers provide alpha-carotene; pumpkin, red peppers and orange-coloured fruit provide cryptoxanthin; tomatoes, particularly processed as in paste or tinned, are the best source of lycopene; leafy greens, such as kale and spinach as well as peas and corn, provide lutein and zeaxanthin; salmon, prawns and other seafood are a good source of astaxanthin	Low-fat diets Artificial fats	
Vitamins E, B3, B6 and C together with magnesium help fats become anti-inflammatory	Fish, nuts, avocado, seeds and their oils	Overheating of foods Saturated fats	

Caring for your joints

One of the most common issues we nutrition consultants deal with is joint pain. In the past, much of the usual advice given by health professionals in relation to diet and joints is quite typical of the One-step Approach in as much as people with joint pain are usually recommended to avoid certain foods (typically those in the Nightshade family, such as potatoes, tomatoes and peppers) and to take supplements with anti-inflammatory properties. A Supereating approach takes things one step further by working to optimize the way nutrients behave.

THE STRUCTURE OF JOINTS

There are over 200 bones in the human body, and the joints where they connect allow normal movement. In very simple terms, to stop bones from rubbing against each other, cartilage is present in the joint cavity along with synovial fluid. Cartilage is flexible yet tough, its consistency lying between hard and fluid, and a typical example is the cartilage that makes up the outer ear. The cartilage is lubricated with viscous gel-like synovial fluid, which is akin to egg white in its consistency. Joint care consists of looking after both cartilage and synovial fluid.

The most common condition to affect the joints is arthritis or inflammation of the substances in the joint cavity. There are two distinct types – rheumatoid arthritis and osteoarthritis. The latter is usually linked to age, typically found in older people whose joints have deteriorated through normal wear and tear, whereas rheumatoid arthritis can affect younger people and is far more associated with inflammation of the joints. Osteoarthritis is typified by a reduction in the cartilage in the joint cavity, leaving the remnants prone to further degradation as they come under increased pressure from the bones, made worse as the area becomes dehydrated.

In the case of rheumatoid arthritis, the synovial fluid is affected, making joints less flexible. As this type of arthritis is considered to be an autoimmune condition, i.e. linked to the immune system not differentiating between 'self' and 'non-self', so increased levels of the typical mediators of inflammation are commonly found. Rheumatoid arthritis is so closely linked to the immune system, it is worth looking at 'Boosting the Immune System' on pages 106–111.

Synovial fluid is made largely from hyaluronic acid (HA), which is itself largely dependent upon magnesium. Cartilage is made from proteoglycans, a substance partially made from HA. Collagen is also a major component, which itself is dependent upon vitamin C for its formation. Keratin is also present and this is reliant on an amino acid found in protein foods, but primarily on sulphur.

INFLAMMATION AND JOINT CARE

Both types of arthritis involve inflammation to one degree or another, and a nutritional approach can help limit the inflammatory response. Two substances, cytokines and prostaglandins, are closely linked to inflammation and both have links to nutrition.

Prostaglandins are derived from fats, more precisely from the essential fats such as omega-3 and -6. The fats we eat are deconstructed and converted into various different fats, ultimately producing one of three types of prostaglandins (PGEs). PGE1 and 3 are considered to have anti-inflammatory effects, while PGE2 can increase inflammation.

In order for omega-3 and -6 fats to be successfully converted into PGE1 or PGE3, specific enzymes are required, known as delta 5 and delta 6 desaturase. To a large degree, these are nutrient-dependent, and require vitamins B3, B6, C and biotin, together with the minerals zinc and magnesium.

Both polyphenols and bioflavonoids are believed to have anti-inflammatory effects as they have an ability to regulate cytokine production. Cytokines are hormone-like substances involved in cell communication as they bind to receptors on the cell and cause a reaction that can increase the inflammatory response (essential in the correct amounts, yet excess is linked to chronic inflammation).

Nutrients for joint health

As both types of arthritis affect synovial fluid and cartilage, the Supereating approach focuses on nutritional approaches to supporting and promoting the production of both of these substances, together with anti-inflammatory measures.

nutrients and their role

Vitamin B3 is required to help derive PGE1 and PGE3 from dietary fats

Vitamin B6 is also required to help derive PGE1 and PGE3 from dietary fats

Vitamin C is required to create anti-inflammatory prostaglandins, and is also a major component of collagen and cartilage

Biotin is required to help derive PGE1 and PGE3 from dietary fats

Zinc is required to help derive PGE1 and PGE3 from dietary fats

Magnesium is involved in the relaxation of the heart muscle and is also required to help control blood pressure

Essential fats with their inherent vitamin E content are the building blocks of anti-inflammatory prostaglandins

Sulphur is a major component of synovial fluid

A day's Supereating

BREAKFAST
plain yoghurt with pumpkin seeds and cantaloupe melon

MORNING SNACK
oatcake with hummus

LUNCH
soft-boiled egg with salad leaves and mushrooms

AFTERNOON SNACK
slice of Cheddar cheese on a rice cake, with ginger tea

DINNER
grilled chicken with onion and garlic dressing, served with cabbage, beans and peas

✔ Friends	*foods to go for*	✘ Foes	*foods to avoid*
Vitamin B6 and iron help release vitamin B3 from tryptophan Other B vitamins	High-protein foods, such as poultry, fish, red meat and liver; chestnut mushrooms; foods high in tryptophan will help boost levels, so dairy foods and eggs would be good choices	Low-protein diets, as amino acids are required to help release B3 Excess cooking	• **Phytate levels**: grain intake should be limited to manage • **Raw vegetables** (steamed is preferable) • **Oxalic acid** (in soft fruits, quinoa, nuts, berries and beans) • **Nightshade family of vegetables** (such as potatoes, tomatoes, peppers, etc.)
Folic acid Vitamin B12 (B6 is required to help release B12 and B3 metabolism has to be good to make B6 available)	Poultry, red meat and offal (particularly liver); pulses (particularly chickpeas); fish; green veg (particularly spinach), asparagus, avocados, cauliflowers, peppers and chestnut mushrooms; root vegetables, leeks and onions; bananas and cantaloupe; cooking with turmeric and ginger (anti-inflammatories) could also improve levels	Cooking and, especially, freezing foods High levels of acid (i.e. vinegar or the like) during cooking	
Bioflavanoids	All fresh fruit and vegetables	Excessive liquid intake Cooking	
Other B vitamins Probiotics	Offal (particularly liver); fish; egg yolk and soya products; nuts (notably hazelnuts); Swiss chard, sweet potato, tomatoes, carrots and avocados	Poor levels of probiotics Raw eggs reduce biotin levels	
Vitamin B6 Cysteine, an amino acid in proteins	Adequate zinc in soil is necessary for plant uptake, so good sources depend on locale; the most available form comes from protein, like meat, game, liver, eggs and seafood (particularly oysters); cheese, yoghurt, beans, nuts and seeds are good sources, but the zinc is less absorbable	Phytates, mainly in grains Cellulose, in leafy plants, so less raw veg (steam) Excess intake of calcium, copper or phosphorus Alcohol and refined sugar	
Calcium Vitamin D	Oat bran, brown rice, quinoa, pumpkin and sunflower seeds, whole grains, nuts, lentils and dark green leafy vegetables	Phosphoric acid (in carbonated drinks) Oxalic acid (in soft fruits, quinoa, nuts, berries and beans)	
B6, carotene zinc, magnesium	Nuts, seeds, fish, avocado and oils	Overheating Saturated fats	
An important metabolic pathway using sulphur is heavily dependent on folate, vitamins B6 and B12	Many foods are good sources of sulphur, including all meat, poultry, eggs and fish; vegetable sources include onions, garlic, cabbage, Brussels sprouts, beans and peas	As mostly found in amino acids, a vegan diet or one low in animal protein may be low in sulphur. High levels of zinc	

Foods for
Supereating

YOU MAY WELL HAVE SEEN LISTS OF FOODS such as this before, indeed I identified the 100 Top Foods in my first book, *The Food Doctor*, published in 1999. The traditional approach has been to show which nutrients are in a food and highlight the benefits for health concerns. Taking this further with Supereating has been a fascinating and worthwhile exercise, as some foods work especially well together, and it is in these combinations that we can really make what we eat work so much more effectively for us.

As nutrition is often full of negative messages, the positive approach of Supereating is a refreshing change. The traditional message of eating plenty of fresh fruits and vegetables, lean protein, essential fats, fibre and water still stands. However, it seems like a natural progression to ask if some fruits or vegetables are more effective than others and as we eat foods in combinations, then how do those foods and the nutrients they contain interact? By using this chapter and the chart on pages 94–7, you should be able to build a food plan of your own as well, and perhaps highlight how you might improve on something that you already do.

For example, if you eat cashew nuts, then you could maximize your uptake of vitamin K by eating them with a probiotic food. This could mean having miso soup alongside your chicken and cashew nuts, or a spoonful of plain yoghurt if you were having the nuts as a snack. Throughout this chapter you will see tips and advice on how to get more from the food you eat, enhancing its benefits.

beans & legumes	vitamins	minerals	other nutrients	Supereating
Adzuki beans	Folic acid Vitamin B1 Vitamin B6	Manganese Phosphorus Potassium	Bioflavonoids Tannins	*All legumes are sources of B vitamins and minerals, and low in fat. They don't need combining with other foods but work best when beans are mixed together for a full range of proteins.*
Chickpeas	Folic acid	Manganese Copper	Bioflavonoids (isoflavones) Saponins (see Grapes)	*A good spread of folate and minerals.*
Kidney beans	Folic acid Vitamin B1	Manganese Iron		*Low in fat and the folate and B1 work well together. Eat with peppers for their vitamin C to enhance iron absorption.*
Lentils	Folic acid Vitamin B1	Manganese Iron	Bioflavonoids (isoflavones)	*Lentils offer 2 complementary B vitamins. Any food rich in vitamin C will enhance iron uptake.*
Mung beans	Folic acid Vitamin B1	Manganese Magnesium Phosphorus	Bioflavonoids	*A source of antioxidants as well as B vitamins, use sprouted seeds for richer source of nutrients.*
Soya beans	Vitamin K Vitamin B2	Manganese Iron	Phyto-oestrogens Saponins (see Grapes)	*Rich in hormone-balancing substances known as phyto-oestrogens. Help the vitamin K absorption by eating with a small amount of any food containing an essential fat, perhaps fish.*
Tofu	Vitamin B1	Manganese Iron Selenium	Omega-3 Phyto-oestrogens	*A rare source of omega-3 for vegetarians. Eat with a food rich in vitamin C to maximize iron uptake and counteract the phytate content.*

eggs & dairy	vitamins	minerals	other nutrients	Supereating
Eggs	Vitamin B2 Vitamin B12 Biotin	Selenium Iodine Phosphorus		*Avoid eating raw (as in steak tartare) as yolk can reduce biotin levels. Selenium and iron are considered to have a positive effect on each other.*
Goats' milk	Vitamin B2	Calcium Phosphorus		*Useful alternative to cows' milk. Having with cereal fortified with vitamin D helps calcium synthesis.*
Yoghurt	Vitamin B2 Vitamin B12	Iodine Calcium Phosphorus	Probiotic bacteria	*The best daily source of probiotics, which help release B vitamins, magnesium, iron and calcium from foods.*
Cottage cheese	Vitamin B12 Vitamin B2	Phosphorus Selenium		*Low-fat cheese, useful source of protein and non-meat source of B12, enhanced by presence of B2, so good for vegetarians.*
Cows' milk	Vitamin D Vitamin B2	Iodine Calcium	Conjugated linoleic acid Omega-3	*Milk is a useful addition to most diets as the calcium is especially easily absorbed. CLA is an excellent antioxidant. Organic milk is a great source of omega-3 fats.*
Feta cheese	Vitamin B2 Vitamin B12	Calcium Phosphorus	Omega-3 Conjugated linoleic acid (CLA, see Cows' milk)	*Feta cheese should be used sparingly as it has a high fat content. It is made from goats' and ewes' milk, so is excellent for those avoiding cows' milk. A good source of B12 for vegetarians and enhanced by the presence of B2.*
Mozzarella	Vitamin B2	Calcium Phosphorus		*Calcium and phosphorous are 'friends', so work well together. Mozzarella can be made from cows' or buffaloes' milk.*

fruit	vitamins	minerals	other nutrients	Supereating
Apples	Vitamin C	Magnesium Calcium	Bioflavonoids (quercetin & kaempferol)	*Low in fructose and high in vitamin C, so useful for helping iron absorption.*
Apricots	Beta-carotene (see Vitamin A and Carotenoids) Vitamin C	Potassium	Carotenoids (lycopene)	*Rich in potent antioxidants. Best eaten with some fat, such as plain almonds, to enhance absorption of carotenoids.*
Bananas	Vitamin B6 Vitamin C	Potassium Manganese	FOS (see right)	*A source of FOS, a prebiotic that helps probiotics thrive and is thus useful for B vitamin and mineral absorption.*
Blackberries	Vitamin C Vitamin K	Manganese Copper	Bioflavonoids (anthocyanins) Carotenoids (lutein & zeacanthin)	*Eat with a source of fat such as a few seeds to help the absorption of vitamin K.*
Blueberries	Vitamin C Vitamin E	Manganese	Bioflavonoids (anthocyanins) Resveratrol (see Other Phytochemicals)	*Rich in antioxidants; eat with some fat such as plain yoghurt or a few nuts to help the absorption of vitamin E.*
Cantaloupe melon	Beta-carotene (see Vitamin A and Carotenoids) Vitamin C	Potassium	Carotenoids	*Eat with some fat to help beta-carotene absorption.*
Cherries	Vitamin C Vitamin K	Potassium	Bioflavonoids (anthocyanins)	*Best eaten with a dietary fat to make the most of the vitamin K content.*
Cranberries	Vitamin C	Manganese	Bioflavonoids (proanthrocyanidins) Resveratrol, see Other Phytochemicals)	*Often sweetened, as otherwise tart, so not an ideal fruit, but still a useful source of antioxidants.*

fruit	vitamins	minerals	other nutrients	Supereating
Figs	Vitamin B6 Vitamin K	Potassium Manganese Calcium	Phytosterols Carotenoids (lutein & zeaxanthin)	*A good antioxidant fruit that contains a little fat in the seeds which helps absorption of the vitamin K and carotenoids.*
Grapefruit	Vitamin C Beta-carotene (see Vitamin A and Carotenoids)	Potassium	Bioflavonoids (limonoids, naringenin) Carotenoids (lycopene)	*Excellent antioxidant, low in fructose but not to be eaten at the same time as several medications (like statins), as action of the fruit lowers their effectiveness. Check labels on any medication.*
Grapes	Vitamin C	Potassium Manganese	Bioflavonoids (quercetin) Resveratrol (see Other Phytochemicals) Saponins (see right)	*Saponins are protective agents in the grapes' waxy skin, which dissolve into the wine during fermentation. Saponins are believed to bind to and prevent the absorption of cholesterol, and are also known to settle down inflammation pathways. High in fructose, so match with a protein for blood glucose management.*
Guava	Vitamin C Folic acid	Potassium Copper	Bioflavonoids Carotenoids (lycopene)	*A good mix of potent antioxidants. Eat with any fat to enhance carotenoid absorption.*
Kiwi fruit	Vitamin C	Potassium	Bioflavonoids Carotenoids (lutein & zeaxanthin)	*Rich in vitamin C and other antioxidants. Its seeds supply the fat necessary for carotenoid absorption.*
Lemons /limes	Vitamin C		Bioflavonoids (flavonol glycosides, limonoids)	*The citric acid content helps mineral absorption, so squeezing lemon or lime juice on food, especially vegetables, enhances their nutritional content.*

fruit	vitamins	minerals	other nutrients	Supereating
Mango	Vitamin C Beta-carotene (see Vitamin A and Carotenoids)	Potassium	Carotenoids (lutein, cryptoxanthin)	*A good antioxidant fruit. Have with seeds or plain yoghurt to enhance absorption.*
Nectarines	Beta-carotene (see Vitamin A and Carotenoids) Vitamin C	Potassium	Carotenoids (cryptoxanthin)	*Useful source of antioxidants; get the best from the beta-carotene by having a few seeds or nuts alongside for their essential fat content.*
Oranges	Vitamin C Folic acid	Potassium	Bioflavonoids (hesperetin, naringenin, anthocyanins) Carotenoids	*Hesperetin has been shown to lower high blood pressure as well as cholesterol in animal studies, and to have strong anti-inflammatory properties. Useful for helping iron absorption.*
Papaya	Vitamin C Folic acid Beta-carotene (see Vitamin A and Carotenoids)	Potassium	Carotenoids (lycopene)	*The seeds contain a digestive enzyme, but aren't especially palatable. Overall a good source of antioxidants but, like other fruits, best eaten with a little fat to get the carotenoid absorbed.*
Peaches	Vitamin C Beta-carotene (see Vitamin A and Carotenoids)	Manganese Copper	Carotenoids (lutein & zeaxanthin) Bioflavonoids (quercetin, kaempferol, anthocyanin)	*Contain a wide range of antioxidants. Make the best of beta-carotene by eating with a food containing an essential fat.*
Pears	Vitamin C Vitamin K	Copper	Carotenoids (lutein)	*Low in fructose and a useful source of vitamin K, which requires fat for absorption.*
Pineapple	Vitamin C Vitamin B1	Manganese	Bromelain (see Other Phytochemicals)	*High in fructose. Best eaten away from phytates as they can reduce manganese absorption.*

fruit	vitamins	minerals	other nutrients	Supereating
Plums	Vitamin C Beta-carotene (see Vitamin A and Carotenoids)	Potassium	Bioflavonoids (anthocyanins)	*Antioxidant-rich fruit. Fats will help beta-carotene to be absorbed.*
Pomegranate	Vitamin C Vitamin B5	Potassium	Bioflavonoids (luteolin)	*Rich in antioxidants and vitamins C and B5 complement one another.*
Prunes	Beta-carotene (see Vitamin A and Carotenoids)	Potassium Copper		*Eat with a fat such as plain yoghurt for carotenoid absorption.*
Raspberries	Vitamin C Folic acid Vitamin B2	Manganese Magnesium	Bioflavonoids (anthocyanins)	*A good spread of nutrients that offer several antioxidants. Eat with calcium-rich fruit, such as rhubarb, to help magnesium levels.*
Rhubarb	Vitamin K Vitamin C	Calcium Potassium Manganese	Carotenoids (lutein, zeaxanthin)	*Like many fruits, rhubarb is best eaten with a fat to help absorption of carotenoids and vitamin K. The refined sugar often added to rhubarb can affect magnesium levels in other foods, so sweeten with apple juice instead.*
Strawberries	Vitamin C	Manganese Potassium	Bioflavonoids (anthocyanins)	*Excellent mix of antioxidants. The tiny seeds contain a little fat that helps absorption, but chew well.*
Watermelon	Vitamin C Beta-carotene (see Vitamin A and Carotenoids) Vitamin B6 Vitamin B1	Potassium Magnesium	Carotenoids (lycopene)	*A good source of antioxidants. Have with plain yoghurt for fat-soluble nutrient absorption.*

fish & seafood	vitamins	minerals	other nutrients	Supereating
Anchovies	Vitamin B3 Vitamin B2 Vitamin B12	Selenium Phosphorus Iron	Omega-3	*Often served salted, but this type are not recommended. Plain anchovies are a good addition to salads as their fat helps absorption of antioxidants.*
Cod	Vitamin B6 Vitamin B12	Selenium Phosphorus	Omega-3	*The combination of B6 and B12 complement one another.*
Haddock	Vitamin B12 Vitamin B3	Selenium Phosphorus	Omega-3	*A good source of vitamin B12 and minerals. Generally low in fat, so not an especially rich source of omega-3.*
Halibut	Vitamin B3	Selenium Phosphorus	Omega-3	*Phosphorus works well with vitamin D, so consider having with a sauce with some cheese in it, or have a slice of cheese afterwards.*
Herring	Vitamin D Vitamin B12 Vitamin B6	Selenium Phosphorus Potassium	Omega-3	*A good mix of nutrients that work well together as they are. Eat with chickpeas to help iron release.*
Mackerel	Vitamin B12 Vitamin D	Selenium Phosphorus	Omega-3	*A rich source of omega-3 and vitamin D, so excellent for bone and skin health.*
Oysters	Vitamin B12	Zinc Copper Selenium		*Low in fat. Eat with some rye bread to help B12 work (rye contains B6).*

fish & seafood	vitamins	minerals	other nutrients	Supereating
Pilchards	Vitamin D Vitamin B12	Selenium Phosphorus	Omega-3	*Pilchards contain an excellent range of nutrients that can be enhanced by combining them with a whole grain and an antioxidant (to help the B12 and protect the omega-3), such as brown rice and sweet potato.*
Prawns	Vitamin D	Selenium Iron	Omega-3 Carotenoids (astaxanthin)	*A worthwhile source of antioxidants. Have with a vegetable rich in vitamin C to help iron absorption.*
Salmon	Vitamin D Vitamin B3 Vitamin B12	Selenium Phosphorus Magnesium	Omega-3 Carotenoids (astaxanthin)	*Offers a highly complementary range of nutrients in one food.*
Sardines	Vitamin B12 Vitamin D	Selenium Phosphorus Calcium	Omega-3	*Packed with omega-3 and vitamin D. The calcium content, along with the fats and vitamin D, make it a very good food for overall bone health.*
Scallops	Vitamin B12	Phosphorus Magnesium	Omega-3	*Have with a whole grain to get some B6 to help the B12 work.*
Tuna	Vitamin B3 Vitamin B6 Vitamin B1	Selenium Phosphorus	Omega-3	*A good source of fats, proteins and nutrients. Eat with an iron-rich vegetable or grain, such as spinach and/or quinoa, to help the B3 convert into the usable form of the vitamin.*

herbs & spices	vitamins	minerals	other nutrients	Supereating
Basil	Vitamin K Beta-carotene (see Vitamin A and Carotenoids)	Iron Calcium	Bioflavonoids (orientin & vicenin)	*The bioflavonoids are absorbed along with the oils, making basil a neat parcel on its own. Best eaten fresh. As the whole leaf is edible, use in abundance to benefit from the nutrients.*
Chillies	Beta-carotene (see Vitamin A and Carotenoids) Vitamin C	Potassium Iron	Capsaicin (see Other Phytochemicals)	*Anti-inflammatory, and recent research suggests it could destroy some cancer cells.*
Cinnamon		Manganese Iron Calcium	Polyphenols (see Iron)	*Cinnamon makes insulin more effective, so useful in keeping energy levels consistent. Sprinkle some on breakfast muesli.*
Garlic	Vitamin B6 Vitamin C	Manganese Selenium	Organosulphides	*Crush to release all the potential of the organosulphides. Add to salads to enhance vitamin C and E release.*
Ginger	Vitamin B6	Potassium Magnesium Copper	Bioflavonoids	*Best not eaten with foods rich in manganese, such as oats and nuts, as the copper content is considered a foe.*
Mint	Beta-carotene (see Vitamin A and Carotenoids)	Calcium	Polyphenols Ursolic acid (see right)	*Ursolic acid is anti-inflammatory, so useful in cases of inflammation. Good source of antioxidants, so add to foods to enhance the immune system.*

herbs & spices	vitamins	minerals	other nutrients	Supereating
Oregano	Vitamin K Beta-carotene (see Vitamin A and Carotenoids)	Manganese Copper	Bioflavonoids Carotenoids	*Unusual in that its two main minerals are considered antagonistic to one another but given the amount of oregano one would use in cooking this is not relevant. Eat with a fat to enhance vitamin absorption.*
Parsley	Vitamin K Vitamin C Beta-carotene (see Vitamin A and Carotenoids)	Iron		*While we don't tend to use herbs in large amounts, using parsley in sauces or fresh on salads offers a good range of nutrients. The iron is well absorbed due to the presence of vitamin C and an olive oil dressing enhances absorption of antioxidants.*
Peppermint	Vitamin C	Manganese		*Peppermint may have mild 'anti-cancer' properties. Combined with an iron-rich food, the vitamin C will help the absorption of the mineral.*
Rosemary		Iron Calcium		*Mild antioxidant properties, like all plants. Eat with a food rich in vitamin C, such as peppers, to enhance iron release.*
Turmeric	Vitamin B6	Manganese Iron Potassium		*Turmeric is noted for its immune-boosting properties. The nutrients all work well together but to get the best of the vitamin B6, mix with another food containing B vitamins. In a curry, the presence of foods rich in vitamin C, such as potato, helps iron release.*

HERBS & SPICES | 157

nuts & seeds	vitamins	minerals	other nutrients	Supereating
Almonds	Vitamin E Vitamin B2 Vitamin K	Manganese Magnesium	Omega-6 Carotenoids (lutein) Bioflavonoids Phytosterols	*The skin of the almond contains many flavonols and so best to eat whole almonds instead of the flaked or blanched ones.*
Brazil nuts	Vitamin B1 Vitamin E	Selenium Magnesium Copper	Phytosterols Omega-6	*Excellent source of selenium and essential fats. Useful in salads or with fruit, to assist assimilation of fat-soluble antioxidants.*
Cashews	Vitamin K Folic acid	Copper Magnesium Phosphorus	Omega-6 Carotenoids (lutein) Bioflavonoids (catechins) Phytosterols	*One of the best sources of copper. As cashews contain vitamin K this can be enhanced by eating them with plain yoghurt for its probiotic properties.*
Flaxseeds (linseeds)	Folic acid Vitamin B6	Manganese Magnesium	Omega-3 Lignans	*More easily absorbed when ground as they are notoriously difficult to chew effectively.*
Hazelnuts	Vitamin E Vitamin B1 Vitamin B2 Vitamin B6	Manganese Copper Magnesium	Omega-6 Carotenoids (lutein) Bioflavonoids (catechins) Phytosterols	*A good spread of nutrients that complement one another. Overall an excellent food, despite the 'foes' status of manganese and copper.*
Macadamia nuts	Vitamin B2	Manganese Copper Magnesium	Monounsaturated fats Phytosterols	*These do contain a good spread of nutrients, but the fat content is very high so this nut is a significant source of calories.*
Pecans	Vitamin B2 Vitamin B6	Manganese Copper Zinc Magnesium	Omega-6 Carotenoids (lutein) Bioflavonoids (catechins) Phytosterols	*Like hazelnuts, pecans have a great range of nutrients which work especially well together (with the exception of manganese and copper), but this is relevant only when consumed in large amounts.*

nuts & seeds	vitamins	minerals	other nutrients	Supereating
Pine nuts	Vitamin E	Zinc Manganese	Omega-6 Carotenoids Bioflavonoids Phytosterols	*Rich in a variety of antioxidants. Add to avocado to assist copper release.*
Pistachios	Vitamin B6 Vitamin B1 Folic acid	Copper Manganese Phosphorus	Carotenoids (lutein) Bioflavonoids Phytosterols	*Particularly high in lutein, a carotenoid, making this a good source of antioxidants. Avoid the salted nuts.*
Pumpkin seeds	Vitamin K	Manganese Magnesium Phosphorus Zinc	Phytosterols Omega-3 Omega-6	*These seeds contain a good ratio of nutrients and also make a good seed butter to use as an alternative to nut butters. Have with probiotic yoghurt to enhance vitamin K.*
Sesame seeds	Vitamin B1	Copper Manganese Calcium	Phytosterols Omega-6	*These tiny seeds need to be well chewed to release the nutrients. Avoid eating with raw fish, to help B1 levels.*
Sunflower seeds	Vitamin E Vitamin B1	Manganese Magnesium Copper	Phytosterols Omega-6	*These contain a variety of nutrients that have antioxidant properties, and are a good choice for a snack as the nutrients work well together.*
Walnuts	Folic acid Vitamin B6	Manganese Copper	Omega-3 Bioflavonoids Carotenoids Phytosterols	*Flavonols, manganese and copper together with carotenoids help make walnuts a good source of antioxidants and a useful alternative to fish as a source of omega-3 fats.*

veg	vitamins	minerals	other nutrients	Supereating
Artichokes	Vitamin C Vitamin K Folic acid	Magnesium Manganese	Phyto-oestrogens (lignans)	*Eat with a grain to assist the folate and a fat such as olive oil to ensure better absorption of vitamin K.*
Asparagus	Vitamin K Folic acid Vitamin C	Manganese Potassium	Carotenoids (lutein & zeaxanthin)	*Delicious with a little hollandaise sauce, which will supply the fat to ensure that vitamin K and carotenoids are more usable. Have alongside any iron-rich food as the vitamin C content is useful.*
Aubergines	Vitamin B1	Potassium Manganese	Bioflavonoids (nasunin)	*An excellent antioxidant vegetable, best served lightly cooked to preserve B1 levels.*
Avocados	Vitamin K Folic acid Vitamin B6	Potassium	Oleic acid (see right) Carotenoids (lutein)	*Oleic acid is a monounsaturated fatty acid that plays a role in lowering cholesterol and helps the carotenoid and vitamin K get absorbed.*
Beetroots	Folic acid Vitamin C	Manganese Potassium	Bioflavonoids Carotenoids	*Preferably served plain roasted rather than pickled or sugared. Manganese works well with iron, as does vitamin C.*
Bok choi	Vitamin A Vitamin C Vitamin K	Calcium	Glucosinolates	*The glucosinolates offer some protection from the formation of cancerous cells. Probiotics enhance their uptake, so have a plain yoghurt dressing on the side, which will also help vitamin K absorption.*

veg	vitamins	minerals	other nutrients	Supereating
Broad beans	Vitamin B2 Vitamin B3	Manganese Copper	Bioflavonoids Carotenoids	*The antioxidants in broad beans are best absorbed with a little fat, so eat alongside fish or drizzle with walnut or olive oil.*
Broccoli	Vitamin C Vitamin K Vitamin A	Manganese Potassium	Glucosinolates (indoles and isothiocyanates such as sulphoraphane) Carotenoids (lutein)	*Requires a fat eaten alongside to maximize use of the glucosinolates and vitamins A and K. Plain yoghurt will work well, perhaps with chopped parsley and lemon juice to add in coumarin and citric acid, making it ideal to combat potentially cancerous cells.*
Brussels sprouts	Vitamin K Vitamin C Folic acid	Manganese Potassium	Glucosinolates (indoles and isothiocyanates such as sulphoraphane) Phyto-oestrogens	*Like broccoli, Brussels sprouts are best eaten with a probiotic and a fat.*
Butternut squash	Beta-carotene (see Vitamin A and Carotenoids) Vitamin C	Potassium Manganese	Carotenoids	*An excellent antioxidant vegetable, make into soup and drizzle a little olive oil on the surface to supply fats to help absorption of carotenoids.*
Cabbage	Vitamin K Vitamin C Vitamin B6	Manganese	Glucosinolates	*Probiotics and fat are required to help absorption of the whole range of nutrients.*
Carrots	Beta-carotene (see Vitamin A and Carotenoids) Vitamin K Vitamin C	Potassium	Carotenoids (lycopene) Lignans	*A great source of antioxidants, best eaten raw to reduce nutrient loss. Eat with nuts to supply fats for carotenoid and vitamin K absorption, ideally pine nuts as they contain vitamin E which works synergistically with vitamin C.*

veg	vitamins	minerals	other nutrients	Supereating
Cauliflower	Vitamin C Vitamin K Folic acid	Manganese	Glucosinolates (indoles and isothiocyanates such as sulphoraphane) Phyto-oestrogens Phytosterols	A probiotic sauce made with milk and a little plain yoghurt will make the glucosinolates in cauliflower more effective. Other B vitamins are useful too, which could be found in whole grains, so a cheese sauce with some breadcrumbs on it could be ideal.
Cavolo nero	Vitamin K Beta-carotene (see Vitamin A and Carotenoids)	Manganese Copper	Glucosinalates Bioflavonoids Carotenoids	This needs to be eaten in a meal that contains fats to help absorption of carotenoids and vitamin A.
Celery	Vitamin K Vitamin C Folic acid	Potassium	Coumarins (See Other Phytochemicals)	Coumarins are important for cardiovascular health. Dip celery in hummus to supply saponins (see Grapes), as these can help reduce cholesterol, and EFAs.
Cucumber	Vitamin C	Potassium		Excellent in salads to help iron absorption of the foods eaten alongside.
Endive (chicory)	Vitamin A Vitamin K Folic acid	Manganese Potassium	Bioflavonoids Carotenoids (lutein & zeaxanthin)	This is best eaten raw in a salad with a dressing made from walnut oil for its B vitamin and fat content.
Fennel	Vitamin C Folic acid	Potassium Manganese	Bioflavonoids (rutin, quercitin, and kaempferol glycosides)	Excellent range of nutrients that work well alone, but can help iron-rich foods do their job more effectively, due to the presence of vitamin C and folate.
Green beans	Vitamin K Vitamin C	Manganese Copper	Bioflavonoids	Eat with a fat, such as flaked almonds or an olive oil dressing, to help vitamin K be utilized.
Jerusalem artichokes	Vitamin B1 Vitamin C Vitamin B3	Iron Potassium	Fructo-oligosaccharides (FOS, see Bananas)	A good source of a prebiotic that helps feed good bacteria in the digestive system. The nutrients complement one another, especially iron and vitamin C.

veg	vitamins	minerals	other nutrients	Supereating
Kale	Vitamin K Beta-carotene (see Vitamin A and Carotenoids)	Manganese Copper	Glucosinalates Bioflavonoids (kaempferol) Carotenoids (lutein and zeaxanthin)	*Powerful anti-cancer properties due to glucosinalates, flavonoids and carotenoids. A probiotic will enhance this, as will Jerusalem artichoke for the prebiotics, so mix together in a salad or eat steamed alongside poultry or fish.*
Kohlrabi	Vitamin C Vitamin B6	Potassium Copper	Bioflavonoids Organosulphides (dithiolthiones and isothiocyanates) Coumarins (See Other Phytochemicals)	*This offers a good range of nutrients and should be eaten away from zinc-rich foods as they can compete for absorption.*
Leeks	Vitamin C Vitamin B6	Manganese Iron	Allium compounds	*Has anti-cancerous properties and can reduce LDL ('bad') cholesterol. The iron and vitamin C complement one another.*
Lettuce	Vitamin K Beta-carotene	Manganese	Carotenoids	*Mostly water, so useful for hydration. The carotenoids require fat for absorption, so eat in a salad with an oil-based dressing and add lemon juice to enhance mineral utilization.*
Lettuce (cos)	Vitamin K Beta-carotene (see Vitamin A and Carotenoids) Vitamin C	Manganese Chromium Potassium	Carotenoids (lutein & zeaxanthin)	*Good antioxidant food, best not eaten with vitamin K foods as chromium can compete for absorption. A fat (oily or creamy dressing) is required, however.*
Mushrooms	Vitamin B2 Vitamin B3	Copper Selenium		*Mushrooms, especially shiitake, are the subject of ongoing research into anti-cancer properties. Remember that mushrooms are a fungus / spore and so not ideal for those who experience bloating or abdominal distension due to wind.*
Okra	Vitamin K Vitamin C	Manganese Magnesium	Carotenoids (lutein & zeaxanthin)	*Eat with a fat to help vitamin and antioxidant absorption.*

veg	vitamins	minerals	other nutrients	Supereating
Onions	Vitamin C Vitamin B6	Chromium Manganese	Allium compounds Bioflavonoids (quercetin) Isothiocynates	*Like leeks, these have many properties, including containing chromium. This doesn't work well with excess vitamin K, so best not to be eaten with cabbage, kale, spinach or broccoli, for example.*
Parsnips	Folic acid Vitamin C	Potassium Manganese	Bioflavonoids Carotenoids	*This needs an essential fat for antioxidant absorption, so roast and then drizzle with a nut or olive oil, but do not cook in oil.*
Peas	Vitamin K Vitamin C Vitamin B1	Manganese	Bioflavonoids Phyto-oestrogens	*A good source of antioxidants but adding a small drizzle of extra virgin olive oil on the top will enable the vitamin K to become absorbed.*
Peppers	Vitamin C Beta-carotene (see Vitamin A and Carotenoids)		Carotenoids (lycopene, lutein, zeaxanthin)	*Rich in a variety of antioxidants, once again a fat is required to enhance absorption.*
Potatoes	Vitamin C Vitamin B6	Copper Potassium Manganese	Carotenoids Bioflavonoids	*Versatile and popular; best eaten with the skin to maximize fibre intake, and alongside fish for essential fat content.*
Pumpkin	Beta-carotene (see Vitamin A and Carotenoids) Vitamin C	Potassium Copper	Carotenoids	*Roast and then sprinkle with cinnamon to help insulin and thus blood glucose; add a little olive oil for absorption.*
Radishes	Vitamin C Folic acid	Potassium	Bioflavonoids	*Eat with a grain for other B vitamins for best folate uptake.*
Sea vegetables	Vitamin K Folic acid	Iodine Magnesium Iron	Lignans	*A good source of iodine, have with a grain such as millet or quinoa, as the iodine will help the B vitamins, especially B3.*

veg	vitamins	minerals	other nutrients	Supereating
Shiitake mushrooms	Vitamin C	Iron Selenium Chromium	Lentinan (increases immune system) Eritadenine (lowers cholesterol) L-ergothioneine (antioxidant)	*Avoid vitamin K foods in same meal; otherwise a good range of nutrients, especially for immune and cardiovascular systems.*
Spinach	Vitamin K Beta-carotene (see Vitamin A and Carotenoids)	Manganese Magnesium	Bioflavonoids Carotenoids (lutein and zeaxanthin)	*Very rich in antioxidants, with 13 different types identified. Have with some olive oil to help absorption.*
Sweet potatoes	Beta-carotene (see Vitamin A and Carotenoids) Vitamin C	Manganese Copper	Carotenoids	*Good antioxidant powers, especially nice eaten raw, grated into salads. Combine with sunflower or pumpkin seeds for fat and mineral content.*
Swiss chard	Vitamin K Beta-carotene (see Vitamin A and Carotenoids) Vitamin C	Magnesium Manganese Potassium	Bioflavonoids (anthocyans) Carotenoids (lutein & zeaxanthin)	*This requires a fat for absorption, so eat alongside fish or poultry.*
Tomatoes	Vitamin C Vitamin K	Potassium	Carotenoids (lycopene)	*Processed tomato contains easily absorbed lycopene, so tomato paste is a good addition to cooking. Eat with a fat.*
Turnips	Vitamin C Vitamin B6 Folic acid	Calcium Potassium	Phytosterols Glucosinalates	*A probiotic enhances the benefits, so when eating turnip, start with a salad with a yoghurt dressing.*
Watercress	Vitamin K Vitamin A Vitamin C	Calcium	Carotenoids (lutein & zeaxanthin) Flavonoids (quercetin) Glucosinolates	*Contains a host of nutrients that have potential to reduce spread of cancerous cells. Also contains a good range of complementary nutrients.*
Yams	Vitamin C Vitamin B6	Copper Potassium Manganese		*A good spread of nutrients and some cholesterol-reducing properties.*

rice & grains	vitamins	minerals	other nutrients	Supereating
Amaranth	Folic acid Vitamin B2	Manganese Magnesium Phosphorus	Phytosterols	*Low phytate content does not inhibit iron absorption, so overall an excellent grain.*
Barley	Vitamin B3 Vitamin B1	Selenium Copper Manganese	Beta-glucans (see right)	*Beta-glucans (a substance found in cereal grains) can reduce cholesterol. The B vitamins work well together but the minerals aren't a perfect combination.*
Brown rice	Vitamin B6 Vitamin B1	Manganese Selenium Magnesium	Phyto-oestrogens	*A wonderful food that has several properties ranging from hormone balancing to being an antioxidant. The phytate content of brown rice is high, so accompany with a vegetable rich in vitamin C, such as sweet potato, to counteract this.*
Buckwheat	Vitamin B3 Vitamin B6 Vitamin B5	Manganese Magnesium	Bioflavonoids (rutin) Phyto-oestrogens (lignans)	*More of a grass than a traditional wheat, so not a source of phytates. The nutrients all work nicely together.*
Corn	Vitamin B1 Folic acid Vitamin C	Phosphorus Manganese		*Its B vitamins work well together and it has antioxidant properties. Useful alongside iron-rich foods due to its vitamin C content.*
Couscous	Vitamin B2 Vitamin B1	Selenium	Phyto-oestrogens	*Great for energy boosting as it contains B vitamins. Cook with vegetable or chicken stock to enhance the flavour. Eat with a spoonful of live yoghurt to supply probiotics and thus enhance vitamin B2.*

rice & grains	vitamins	minerals	other nutrients	Supereating
Millet	Vitamin B1 Vitamin B3 Vitamin B6	Manganese Magnesium Phosphorus		*Antioxidant grain with low phytate content. Help the magnesium content by having a food rich in vitamin D at the same meal.*
Oats	Vitamin B1	Manganese Selenium Phosphorus	Beta-glucans (see Barley above) Phyto-oestrogens	*Beta-glucans helps reduce and protect cholesterol. Phytate content is average, but the numerous benefits of oats far outweigh any phytate consideration.*
Quinoa	Vitamin B2 Vitamin B1	Manganese Magnesium	Phyto-oestrogens	*A versatile grain that has a good spread of nutrients. Absorption can be improved if eaten with vitamin D-rich foods.*
Rye	Vitamin B3 Vitamin B1	Manganese Selenium	Phyto-oestrogens	*Low in phytates. Make the minerals work better by eating with an iron-rich food such as sardines.*
Spelt	Vitamin B3 Vitamin B1	Manganese Phosphorus Magnesium	Phyto-oestrogens	*Lower in phytates than regular wheat, spelt flour is a useful alternative.*
Wild rice	Vitamin B3 Vitamin B6 Folic acid	Manganese Zinc		*A grass rather than a rice, it is rich in complementary B vitamins.*
Whole wheat	Vitamin B3 Folic acid	Manganese Magnesium	Phyto-oestrogens	*A source of phytates but this can be compensated for by eating with vitamin-C-rich foods and probiotics (for example, plain yoghurt with parsley somewhere in the same meal).*

poultry & lean meats	vitamins	minerals	other nutrients	Supereating
Chicken	Vitamin B3 Vitamin B6	Selenium Phosphorus		*Without the skin, chicken is a low-fat poultry that offers antioxidants and protein. Have with a side dish of edamame and/or mushrooms to enhance absorption of phosphorus into the bones.*
Pork fillet	Vitamin B1 Vitamin B6 Vitamin B3	Selenium Phosphorus Potassium		*The fat content of pork is higher than poultry, but not as high as traditional red meat, making it a good compromise. A good spread of minerals and B vitamins together with protein. Eat with mushrooms as above.*
Turkey	Vitamin B3 Vitamin B6	Selenium Phosphorus		*Very low in fat, turkey is a useful source of nutrients. Eat with mushrooms or edamame as above.*
Venison	Vitamin B12 Vitamin B2 Vitamin B3	Iron Phosphorus Selenium		*Eat with vegetables containing vitamin C, such as green beans or peas, to help iron uptake. Eat with mushrooms or edamame as above.*

others	vitamins	minerals	other nutrients	Supereating
Green tea			Bioflavonoids (catechin)	*Very rich in antioxidants and low in caffeine.*
Honey			Probiotics	*Some mild antibacterial qualities but, despite the benefits, honey does perpetuate the desire for sweet foods so should be used very occasionally.*
Miso	Vitamin K Vitamin B2	Manganese Zinc Copper	Probiotics	*A good source of probiotics, so useful instead of plain yoghurt when they are called for. Starting a meal with some miso soup is highly beneficial.*
Olive oil	Vitamin E		Omega-6	*Oleic acid is a monounsaturated fatty acid which plays a role in lowering cholesterol. Adding it to any food rich in vitamin C will help recycle and preserve nutrients.*
Spirulina	Beta-carotene (see Vitamin A and Carotenoids) Vitamin B12	Potassium Iron Magnesium	Carotenoids	*A complete protein and very nutrient-dense, but requires a fat eaten with it or in the same meal to help the absorption of carotenoids. A vitamin B6 food will also help the B12, so consider a slice of avocado in the same meal.*

Glossary

Amino acids are the basic components of proteins. There are 20 essential amino acids and the body can only produce half of these (alanine, asparagine, aspartic acid, **cysteine**, glutamic acid, glutamine, glycine, proline, serine and tyrosine) so the others – arginine and **histidine** (required for the young, but not for adults), isoleucine, leucine, lysine, **methionine**, phenylalanine, threonine, **tryptophan**, and valine – must be obtained via food.

Anaemia is a condition caused by a deficiency of **haemoglobin** in the blood so that the organs are deprived of adequate oxygen.

Anthocyanins, part of the flavonoid family, are present to some degree in most plants and are responsible for some of the deep red-blue pigmentation of some fruits and vegetables. They are also potent **antioxidants**.

Anthocyanidins are sugar-free versions of **anthocyanins**, which also have important antioxidant properties.

Antibodies, part of the immune system and also known as immunoglobulins, are proteins found in the blood or other bodily fluids that are used to identify and neutralize foreign objects, such as bacteria and viruses.

Antioxidants are compounds in foods that seek out and neutralize potentially damaging **free radicals** in the body.

Arrhythmia is a general term used for any form of irregular heartbeat.

Ascorbic acid is the chemical name for vitamin C.

Astaxanthin, part of the carotenoid family, are the chemicals that provide the pink or red pigment in fish and shellfish. They are powerful **antioxidants**.

Bifidobacteria are the bacteria that make up a large part of the intestinal flora, aiding digestion and lowering the incidence of allergies.

Bromelain is a mixture of protein-digesting **enzymes** found in pineapples.

Calcitriol is the term for the active form of vitamin D found in the body. It increases the absorption of calcium and phosphate from the **gastrointestinal tract** and kidneys.

Capsaicin is the chemical that gives chillies their heat. Found throughout the pepper, but concentrated mostly in the pale placental membrane around the seeds, it is finding use as a natural local anaesthetic, and research seems to indicate it has powerful anti-cancer properties.

Catechins are the flavonoids found in tea that have powerful antioxidant properties.

Chrohn's disease is a disorder of the **gastrointestinal (GI) tract** in which its lining becomes inflamed, most commonly in the lower part of the small intestine.

Cobalamin is the chemical name for vitamin B12.

Coeliac Disease is an autoimmune disease in which the body's immune system attacks its own tissues, which is triggered by gluten, a collective name for a type of protein found in the cereals wheat, rye and barley. A few people are also sensitive to oats. Eating gluten causes the lining of the gut (small bowel) to become damaged.

Coenzymes are small organic non-protein molecules that carry chemical groups between **enzymes**.

Coenzyme A is a **coenzyme** present in all living cells, which is essential to metabolism of carbohydrates and fats and some **amino acids**.

Collagen is the major protein component of the connective tissue and constitutes about 25% to 35% of the total protein in mammals. Collagen molecules have remarkably diverse forms and functions. For example, collagen in tendons forms stiff, rope-like fibres of tremendous tensile strength; while in skin, collagen takes the form of loosely woven fibres, permitting expansion in all directions.

Coumarin is a phytochemical that has a vanilla-like flavour and is responsible for the sweet smell of new-mown hay. It is found in several plants, including tonka beans, lavender, licorice, strawberries, apricots, cherries, cinnamon and sweet clover, and seems to have blood-thinning, anti-fungicidal and anti-tumour properties.

Cryptoxanthin is one of the carotenoid family of phytochemicals, and is another plant pigment with **antioxidant** properties. In the body it is converted into vitamin A.

Cysteine is a non-essential **amino acid**; this is one of the few amino acids to contain sulphur and has an important role in the immune system as well as in protecting the linings of the stomach and intestines.

Egosterol is the compound in our skin that converts sunshine into vitamin D. It is also found in some plants.

Electrolytes are salts found in the body fluid, tissue, and blood that conduct electricity and are essential for muscle coordination, heart function, fluid absorption and excretion, nerve function and concentration.

Enzymes are types of proteins that act as catalysts, initiating, speeding up or slowing down chemical reactions in the body.

Flavanols are a type of flavonoid, mostly found in cocoa and chocolate, tea and wine, and are thought to be linked to a range of circulatory health benefits.

Flavones are types of flavonoids, most commonly found in celery and parsley, and responsible for the yellowish component of their pigment.

Folate is the term for the chemical form of folic acid (vitamin B9) when found in plants and our bodies.

Free radicals are atoms or groups of atoms with an odd (unpaired) number of electrons and can be formed when oxygen interacts with certain molecules. These highly reactive radicals can start a chain reaction, but the greatest damage they can do is when they react with important cellular components such as DNA, or the cell membrane. Such cells may then function poorly or die. **Antioxidants** are the best means of neutralizing **free radicals** and the damage they cause.

Fructose is the simple sugar found in fruits, honey and sweet vegetables like carrots.

Gastrointestinal tract (**GI**) is the term for the passageway that starts with the mouth and proceeds to the esophagus, stomach, duodenum, small intestine, large intestine (colon), rectum and, finally, the anus.

Glucose is the principal simple sugar and the form in which sugar circulates in the blood, to be used by the metabolism to provide us with energy.

Glutathione peroxidase is an **enzyme** in the body that is a powerful scavenger of **free radicals**.

Glutathione, also known as GSH, is the most powerful naturally occurring **antioxidant** in all human cells. It also plays a major part in the immune system, having a critical role in the multiplication of lymphocytes.

Haemoglobin is the iron-containing protein attached to red blood cells that transports oxygen from the lungs to the rest of the body. Haemoglobin bonds with oxygen in the lungs, exchanges it for carbon dioxide at cellular level, and then transports the carbon dioxide back to the lungs to be exhaled.

Haemochromatosis is an hereditary disease, most prevalent among northern Europeans, makes the body absorb too much iron, which can damage the major organs like the liver and the heart.

Hesperedin is a bioflavonoid found in citrus peel that inhibits the release of histamine, thus reducing allergic reactions and the symptoms of asthma. It also helps control blood cholesterol levels and has

antioxidant and anti-inflammatory properties.

Histidine is an amino acid that is particularly important in the protection of tissue, especially the myelin sheath that protects the nerves.

Homocysteine is a form of the **amino acid cysteine**, high levels of which are increasingly being held to be an important factor in cardiovascular disease.

Hydroxyapatite is a naturally occurring form of the mineral calcium apatite is one of the prime constituents of bones and teeth.

Hypercalcaemia is the medical term for very elevated levels of calcium in the blood. As it is often an indication of major problems, particularly cancer, it is usually a matter of concern.

Indole-3-carbinol, produced by the breakdown of the glucosinolate glucobrassicin (found at relatively high levels in cruciferous vegetables) is the subject of on-going research into its possible anticarcinogenic and **antioxidant** effects.

Inositol, found in grains, beans, nuts and fruit, performs important functions in the body, notably in breaking down fats, lowering blood cholesterol and keeping the nervous system healthy. At one time it was classified as vitamin B8, but when it was later discovered that the body could synthesize it, it was declassified.

Irritable bowel syndrome (**IBS**) is a common gut disorder. The cause is not known. Symptoms can include abdominal pain, bloating, and sometimes bouts of diarrhoea and/or constipation.

Insulin is a hormone that causes most of the body's cells to take up glucose from the blood, storing it as glycogen in the liver and muscle, and stops use of fat as an energy source. When insulin is absent (or low), **glucose** is not taken up by most body cells and the body begins to use stored fat as an energy source. When control of insulin levels fails, diabetes results.

Intrinsic factor is a protein secreted in the gastric juices, which is required for the absorption of vitamin B12; lower levels can result in pernicious **anaemia**.

Inulins are a group of naturally occurring polysaccharides (several simple sugars linked together) used by some plants as a means of storing energy and typically found in roots or rhizomes. The food processing industry make great use of inulins to replace sugar, fat and flour, particularly as they contain a third to a quarter of the food energy of sugar or other carbohydrates and a sixth to a ninth of the food energy of fat. Inulins also increase calcium absorption and possibly magnesium absorption, while promoting the growth of intestinal bacteria.

Isoflavones, related to the flavonoids, are organic compounds most commonly found in soy products, which are strong **antioxidants** and act as phyto-oestrogens.

Isothiocyanates are a group of phytochemicals termed glucosinolates that are found in plants and cruciferous vegetables, such as watercress, Brussels sprouts, broccoli, cabbage, kai choi, kale, horseradish, radish and turnip. In many research trials they have been found to inhibit the development of tumours and are being investigated as possible preventive agents for specific human cancers.

Keratin is an extremely strong protein, which is a major component in skin, hair, nails, and teeth. The amino acids that make up keratin have several unique properties, and depending on the levels of the various amino acids, keratin can be inflexible and hard, like horses' hooves, or soft, as is the case with human skin.

Lactobacilli are one of the types of friendly bacteria present in the gut flora. They convert sugars into lactic acid, which helps produce an environment that discourages growth of unfriendly bacteria.

Lignans are a major group of phyto-oestrogens and strong antioxidants that are found in greatest quantity in flax and sesame seeds, but also in soy products, cereals like oats and barley, and some vegetables, like broccoli.

Lipid is a broad chemical term for naturally occurring molecules that are soluble in fat and includes most of what we normally think of as fats, the essential fatty acids, fat-soluble vitamins, steroids, cholesterol, etc.

Lutein is one of the many carotenoids, and is primarily found in green leafy vegetables such as spinach and kale. Lutein is an antioxidant and is thought to have beneficial effects on both the skin and the eyes.

Lycopene, a carotenoid, is the red pigment in tomatoes and is one of the most potent antioxidants in that huge family. It has also been found to maintain its powers even when the tomatoes are cooked or processed.

Malic acid is the compound responsible for the sour taste in many foods, especially unripe fruit. It is a key chemical in the Kreb's cycle of energy creation from food in the body.

Menaquinone is a form of Vitamin K produced by the intestinal flora. It plays an important part in blood coagulation.

Methionine is one of the essential **amino acids**; it plays an essential part in the breakdown of fats, detoxifying the liver and building muscle tissue. Its best sources include seeds, nuts, fish and meats.

Naringin is the flavonoid present in citrus fruit, especially the grapefruit, which gives it a bitter flavour. As well a being a potent **antioxidant**, it is also thought to have possible anti-cancer properties.

Nicotinamide is the chemical term for a form of vitamin B3.

Osteomalacia is the general term for the softening of the bones due to insufficient mineral absorption, which is know in children as rickets.

Osteoporosis, or brittle bone disease, is a disease of the bones, most common in post-menopausal women, in which the bone mineral density is reduced, leading to an increased risk of fracture.

Oxalates are salts or esters of oxalic acid that bind themselves to minerals, such as calcium and iron, so that they cannot be absorbed by the body. Moreover, kidney stones are mostly calcium oxalate. The irony is that oxalates are found in a wide range of otherwise very healthy and nutritious foods, such as spinach, chard, blackberries and tofu, to name but a few.

Pantothenic acid is the chemical term for vitamin B5.

Pathogens are any biological agent that can cause disease or illness.

Phosphates are salts or esters of phosphoric acid. Diets high in phosphates, such as carbonated drinks and other soft drinks, as well as processed foods (in which they are used for their preservative qualities) may have a deleterious effect on calcium absorption.

Phospholipids are types of lipids containing **phosphates** that are used in the formation of biological membranes such as those of our bodies' cells.

Phylloquinone is the chemical term for the form of vitamin K found in food.

Phytates are salts of phytic acid, found in the hulls of nuts, seeds and grains, where they are the principal means of storing phosphorus. Although they are strongly **antioxidant**, they have the very negative effect of binding up minerals like magnesium, calcium, iron and zinc, so that the body cannot absorb them.

Phytosterol, or plant sterols, perform the same function in plants' cell membranes as cholesterol does in mammals. In the human body they have the effect of lowering blood cholesterol levels.

Polyphenols are chemicals found in plants that have several basic forms: two of which, **tannins** and **flavonoids** are of note in our context. Polyphenols were once briefly known as vitamin P, but were subsequently found non-essential and declassified.

Prebiotics are generally any food or drink that can increase the number and/or activity of **bifidobacteria** and lactic acid bacteria in the gut.

Prostaglandins are compounds derived from essential fatty acids that have an amazing array of powers of control over many of the body's functions, from controlling cell growth and hormones to maintaining the smooth contraction and expansion of the bowels.

Pyridoxine is the chemical term for one of the compounds known as Vitamin B6.

Quercetin is among the most active of the flavonoids and many medicinal plants owe much of their activity to their high quercetin content. It has significant anti-inflammatory properties and inhibits both the manufacture and release of histamine and other allergic/inflammatory mediators. In addition, it exerts potent **antioxidant** activity and several studies show it has anti-tumour properties.

Resveratrol is a natural antibiotic produced by several plants when under attack by bacteria or fungi. It is most commonly found in Japanese knotweed, in the skin and seeds of red grapes (and thus red wine), in peanuts, cranberries and other berry fruit. It has been the subject of many interesting studies in several areas and appears to extend the life of small animals, display anti-cancer properties and aid athletic endurance.

Retinoids is the term for the various compounds that make up vitamin A.

Riboflavin is the chemical term for vitamin B2.

Rutin is a flavonoid related to **hesperidin** and found principally in apricots, buckwheat, cherries, prunes, rose hips, the whitish rind of citrus fruits, and the core of green peppers, that as well as being a powerful **antioxidant** also acts to strengthen the capillaries and to lower LDL (bad) cholesterol levels in the blood.

Salicylates occur naturally in many plant foods, notably the bark of the willow tree and the herb meadowsweet, acting as plant hormones. They have long been known to have significant anti-fever, anti-inflammatory and pain relief properties, as well as helping with warts and other skin problems. The compounds are also manufactured synthetically and used to make painkilling drugs, such as aspirin and ibuprofen, as well as artificial flavourings, skin care products and preservatives.

Saponins are a group of bitter-tasting substances that occur in plants and can produce a soapy lather with water. Extracted commercially from soapwort, they are used as foam producer in beverages and for emulsifying oils.

Sebum is the oily secretion of the sebaceous glands that acts to protect and waterproof hair and skin, and keep them from becoming dry, brittle, and cracked. It can also inhibit the growth of microorganisms on the skin.

Sterols, *see* phytosterols

Superoxide dismutase, or SOD, is a naturally **antioxidant enzyme** present in the human body in three forms: SOD1 is located in the cytoplasm (the fluid within cells), SOD2 in the mitochondria (the cells' power sources) and SOD3 is extracellular. SOD1 and SOD3 contain copper and zinc, while SOD2 has manganese. SOD forms the body's own front line against **free radical** damage.

Tannins are the plant **polyphenols** that give things like red wine, tea and unripe fruit the bitter component of their flavour. They can have many positive effects, including wound and burn healing and acting as anti-inflammatories, but they do have the very negative effect of binding metallic minerals, like iron and zinc, so that the body cannot absorb them.

Tartaric acid is a natural acid found in many plants, notably grapes, bananas and tamarind, which has **antioxidant** properties and is used in food processing as a preservative.

Thiamine is the chemical term for vitamin B1.

Thymus is the gland located between the lungs and behind the sternum, which produces hormones essential in the making of the immune system's T cells.

Thyroid is the gland found in the neck that controls how quickly the body burns energy, makes proteins, and controls how sensitive the body should be to other hormones.

Tocopherols and **tocotrienols** are chemical compounds, eight of which constitute vitamin E. Alpha-tocopherol is the form of vitamin E that is preferentially absorbed and accumulated in humans.

Tryptophan is one of the essential **amino acids,** necessary for normal growth in infants and for nitrogen balance in adults. It is also involved in healthy brain chemistry and is claimed to be a natural anti-depressant. Found in most protein-based foods or dietary proteins, it is particularly plentiful in chocolate, oats, bananas, mangoes, dried dates, milk, yogurt, cottage cheese, red meat, eggs, fish, poultry, sesame, chickpeas, sunflower seeds, pumpkin seeds and peanuts.

Zeaxanthin is a carotenoid that is almost exactly the same as **lutein** and has the same **antioxidant** powers and benefits for eye and skin health.

Index

First published in 2008 by
Quadrille Publishing Limited,
Alhambra House,
27–31 Charing Cross Road,
London WC2H 0LS

Editorial Director: Jane O'Shea
Creative Director: Helen Lewis
Editor and Project Manager: Lewis Esson
Art Director: Ros Holder
Photography: William Reavell
Production Director: Vincent Smith
Production Controller: Ruth Deary

Cataloguing in Publication data: a catalogue reference for this book is available from the British Library.

ISBN 978 184400 628 1

Printed and bound in China

Acknowledgements

With grateful thanks to my lovely new publishers, Quadrille,
especially Alison Cathie and Jane O'Shea, and to my editor
Lewis Esson for his valuable input and guidance. Rowena Paxton
for her willingness to travel and her dedicated research. Special
thanks to all my colleagues at The Food Doctor, especially Erika
Andersson for her unending support and Lisa Blair for her
research skills.

The publishers would like to thank Katherine Case for art
directing the photography, Nicola Davidson for design assistance,
and Simon Davis for editorial assistance.

The research that supports the Supereating approach is available
at www.thefooddoctor.com